ULTIMATE KETO COOKBOOK

KETO MAGIC!

The Only Ketogenic Cookbook You Will Ever Need Packed With Keto Meal Plan, Delicious Keto Recipes, Proven Meal Prep For Two with Anti-Inflammatory Recipes

SAMMY FAY

Copyright © 2020 Sammy Fay

All Rights Reserved

Copyright 2020 By Sammy Fay - All rights reserved.

The following book is produced below with the goal of providing information that is as accurate and reliable as possible. Regardless, purchasing this eBook can be seen as consent to the fact that both the publisher and the author of this book are in no way experts on the topics discussed within and that any recommendations or suggestions that are made herein are for entertainment purposes only. Professionals should be consulted as needed prior to undertaking any of the action endorsed herein.

This declaration is deemed fair and valid by both the American Bar Association and the Committee of Publishers Association and is legally binding throughout the United States.

Furthermore, the transmission, duplication or reproduction of any of the following work including specific information will be considered an illegal act irrespective of if it is done electronically or in print. This extends to creating a secondary or tertiary copy of the work or a recorded copy and is only allowed with express written consent from the Publisher. All additional right reserved.

The information in the following pages is broadly considered to be a truthful and accurate account of facts and as such any inattention, use or misuse of the information in question by the reader will render any resulting actions solely under their purview. There are no scenarios in which the publisher or the original author of this work can be in any fashion deemed liable for any hardship or damages that may befall them after undertaking information described herein.

Additionally, the information in the following pages is intended only for informational purposes and should thus be thought of as universal. As befitting its nature, it is presented without assurance regarding its prolonged validity or interim quality. Trademarks that are mentioned are done without written consent and can in no way be considered an endorsement from the trademark holder.

Table of Contents

- PART I 10
- Keto Recipes 11
  - Chapter 1: Gourmet Recipes 13
    - Creamy Garlic Chicken 13
    - Mediterranean Lemon Herb Chicken Salad 14
    - Garlic Butter Scallops and Steak 16
    - Fried Chicken 18
    - Lime Chile Steak Fajitas 20
    - Spaghetti Squash With Stuffed Lasagna 22
    - Zucchini Boats With Stuffed Tuna 23
    - Spinach and Goat Cheese Stuffed Breast of Chicken 24
  - Chapter 2: Quick and Easy Recipes 25
    - Antipasto Salad 25
    - Feta Cheese and Chicken Plate 26
    - Cheese Omelet 26
    - Baked Salmon and Pesto 28
    - Pork Chops and Blue Cheese Sauce 30
    - Green Pepper and Pork Stir-Fry 32
    - Broccoli With Fried Chicken 33
    - Fried Eggs With Pork and Kale 34
  - Chapter 3: Sweet Recipes 34
    - Sugar Cinnamon Donuts 35
    - Mug Brownie 37
    - Mini Cheesecake 39
    - Keto Fudge 42
    - Peanut Butter Hearts 43
    - Peanut Butter and White Chocolate Blondies 44

- Low Carb Ice Cream 45
- Chocolate Donut 47
- Chapter 4: Savory Recipes 48
  - Keto McMuffin 48
  - Sausage Hash With Rainbow Chard 50
  - Veggie and Chicken Sausage Skillet 51
  - Cheese and Crispy Salami 52
  - Buffalo Chicken Sandwich 53
  - Cream Cheese and Salmon Bites 54
  - Turkey Patties 57
- Chapter 5: Poultry and Meat Recipes 58
  - Beef Cabbage Skillet 58
  - Meatball Casserole 59
  - Beef Taquitos 61
  - Chicken Wings 62
  - Roasted Leg of Chicken 64
- Chapter 6: Staple Recipes 66
  - Keto Waffles 66
  - Cookie Dough 68
  - Baked Tofu 69
  - Cauliflower Fried Rice 70

PART II 71

Vegan Cookbook 72

- Chapter 1: Breakfast Recipes 74
  - Shamrock Sandwich 74
  - Breakfast Burrito 76
  - Gingerbread Waffles 78
  - Green Chickpeas And Toast 80
  - Asparagus And Tomato Quiche 81

    Breakfast Bowl 83

    Tofu Pancakes 85

Chapter 2: Side Dish Recipes 87

    Baked Beans 87

    Baked Potato Wedges 88

    Black Beans And Quinoa 90

    Roasted Lemon Garlic Broccoli 91

    Spicy Tofu 92

    Spanish Rice 93

    Pepper And Lemon Pasta 94

Chapter 3: High Protein Recipes 95

    Kale Salad With Spicy Tempeh Bits And Chickpeas 95

    Protein Bars 97

    Tofu And Spinach Scramble 99

    Vegan Tacos 100

    Grilled Tofu Steaks And Spinach Salad 102

    Corn, Quinoa, And Edamame Salad 104

    Lentil Soup 105

Chapter 4: Dessert Recipes 107

    Chocolate Pudding 107

    Orange Cake 109

    Pumpkin Tofu Pie 111

    Vegan Brownie 113

    Vegan Cupcake 114

    Vanilla Cake 115

    Miracle Fudge 116

Chapter 5: Sauces & Dips Recipes 118

    Tomato Jam 118

    Walnut Kale Pesto 119

Ranch Dressing 120
PART III 121
Chapter 1: Identifying the Mediterranean Diet 122
    Defining the Mediterranean Lifestyle 122
    The Rules of the Mediterranean Diet 123
Chapter 2: Savory Mediterranean Meals 125
    Mediterranean Feta Mac and Cheese 126
    Chickpea Stew 126
    Savory Mediterranean Breakfast Muffins 127
    Mediterranean Breakfast Bake 128
    Mediterranean Pastry Pinwheels 128
Chapter 3: Sweet Treats on the Mediterranean Diet 130
    Greek Yogurt Parfait 130
    Overnight Oats 131
    Apple Whipped Yogurt 131
Chapter 4: Gourmet Meals on the Mediterranean Diet 133
    Garlic-Roasted Salmon and Brussels Sprouts 133
    Walnut Crusted Salmon with Rosemary 134
    Spaghetti and Clams 135
    Braised Lamb and Fennel 135
    Mediterranean Cod 137
    Baked Feta with Olive Tapenade 138
Chapter 5: 30-Minutes or Less Meals 139
    Vegetarian Toss Together Mediterranean Pasta Salad 139
    Vegetarian Aglio e Olio and Broccoli 139
    Cilantro and Garlic Baked Salmon 141
    Harissa Pasta 142
Chapter 6: 1-Hour-or-Less Meals 143
    1 Hour Baked Cod 143

Grilled Chicken Mediterranean Salad..144

Lemon Herb Chicken and Potatoes One Pot Meal.......................146

Vegetarian Mediterranean Quiche 147

Herbed Lamb and Veggies...148

Chicken and Couscous Mediterranean Wraps 150

Sheet Pan Shrimp..151

Mediterranean Mahi Mahi...153

Chapter 7: Slow Cooker Meals 154

Slow Cooker Mediterranean Chicken..154

Slow Cooker Vegetarian Mediterranean Stew 156

Vegetarian Slow Cooker Quinoa..157

Slow-Cooked Chicken and Chickpea Soup 159

Slow Cooked Brisket..160

Vegan Bean Soup with Spinach..161

Moroccan Lentil Soup 162

Chapter 8: Vegetarian and Vegan Meals 163

Vegetarian Greek Stuffed Mushrooms 163

Vegetarian Cheesy Artichoke and Spinach Stuffed Squash 164

Vegan Mediterranean Buddha Bowl 165

Vegan Mediterranean Pasta...167

Vegetarian Zucchini Lasagna Rolls 169

Vegetarian Breakfast Sandwich..170

Vegan Breakfast Toast...171

Vegetarian Shakshouka 172

PART I

Keto Recipes

The keto diet is a high-fat and low-carb diet that comes with various health benefits. It has been found that this diet can help you lose weight and improve the condition of your health. It might also show some positive effects on cancer, diabetes, Alzheimer's, and epilepsy. This diet's main aim is to reduce the intake of carbs drastically and replace the same with healthy fats. When you reduce the consumption of carbs, the body will enter a metabolic state known as ketosis. During ketosis, the body will try its best to burn the body fat for generating energy. It will also be turning the liver fat into ketones that supply energy to the brain.

A keto diet is a very effective way of losing weight. The best aspect of this diet is that you can lose bodyweight without counting calories. The reason behind this is that the diet will be so filling that you will not have frequent cravings. It has been found that people who follow a keto diet can lose 2.5 times more weight when compared to those people who follow a calorie-restrictive diet. The keto diet can also deal with type 2 diabetes, metabolic, and prediabetes syndrome. Some other benefits of the keto diet are:

- **Cancer:** This diet can help suppress the growth of tumors and might also help in treating various types of cancer.

- **Heart diseases:** The keto diet can help deal with various chronic heart conditions such as heart attack, stroke, and others.

- **Polycystic ovary:** This diet is well known for reducing insulin levels that can help in dealing with polycystic ovary.

There are certain food items that you will need to include while following this diet.

- **Fatty fish**: Trout, salmon, mackerel, tuna

- **Meat**: Steak, sausage, red meat, ham, chicken, bacon, turkey

- **Seeds and nuts**: Walnuts, almonds, pumpkin seeds, flax seeds, chia seeds

- **Oils**: Coconut oil, olive oil, avocado oil

A keto diet is an excellent option for all those who have diabetes, overweight or want to improve the health of their metabolism. I have included some tasty and easy keto recipes that you can include in your diet plan.

Chapter 1: Gourmet Recipes

If you are looking for some tasty keto gourmet recipes, this section has got what you are searching for. So, let's have a look at them.

Creamy Garlic Chicken

Total Prep & Cooking Time: Twenty-five minutes

Yields: Six servings

Nutrition Facts: Calories: 348 | Protein: 28g | Carbs: 6.3g | Fat: 22.3g | Fiber: 0.9g

Ingredients

- Two pounds of chicken breasts (sliced thinly)
- Two tbsps. of olive oil
- One cup of each
    - Heavy cream
    - Spinach (chopped)
- Half cup of each
    - Chicken stock
    - Parmesan cheese
    - Sun-dried tomatoes
- One tsp. of each
    - Italian seasoning
    - Garlic powder

Method:

1. Take an iron skillet and add olive oil in it. After the oil gets hot, add the chicken and cook for five minutes. Remove the pieces of chicken from the skillet. Keep aside.

2. Add chicken stock, heavy cream, Italian seasoning, garlic powder, and parmesan cheese in the skillet. Whisk the mixture on medium flame until the sauce thickens. Add tomatoes and spinach. Simmer the mixture for two minutes until the spinach wilts.

3. Addcooked chicken into the prepared sauce. Cook for two minutes.

4. Serve hot.

Mediterranean Lemon Herb Chicken Salad

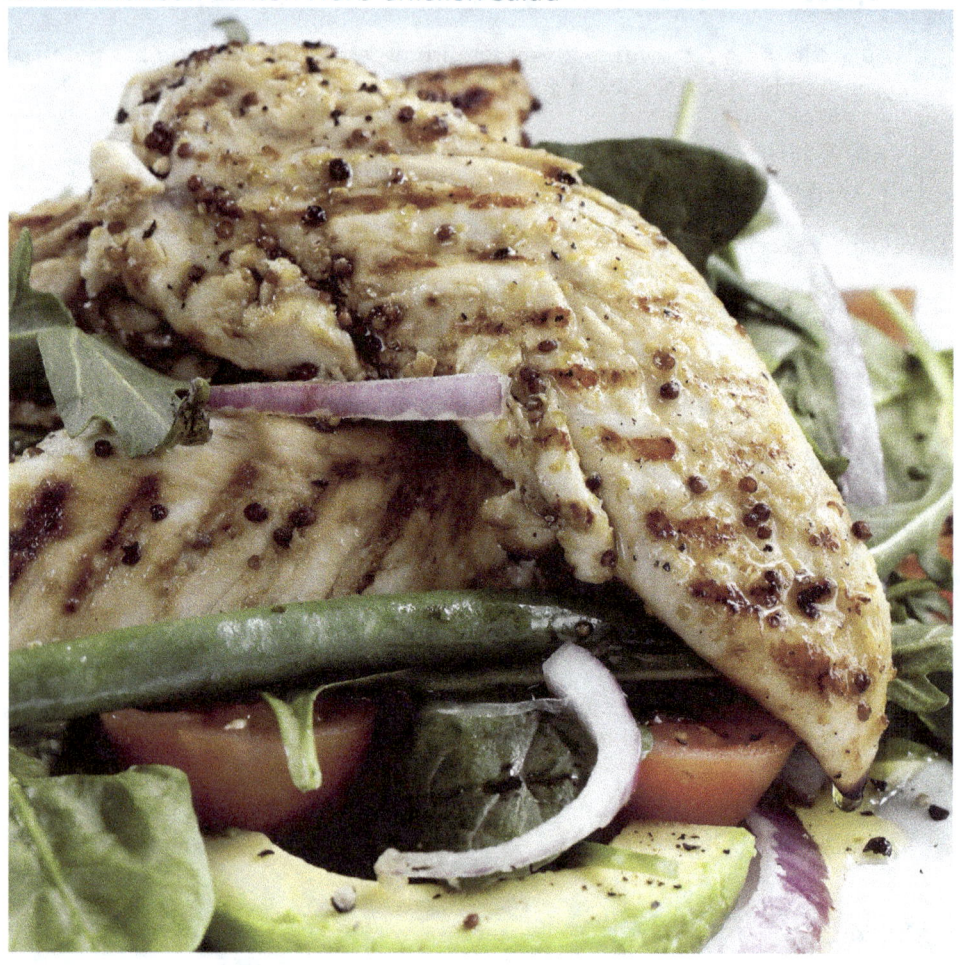

Total Prep & Cooking Time: Twenty-five minutes

Yields: Four servings

Nutrition Facts: Calories: 326 | Protein: 22.3g | Carbs: 12g | Fat: 20.1g | Fiber: 6.2g

Ingredients

- Two tbsps. of each
    - Olive oil
    - Water
    - Parsley (chopped)
    - Red wine vinegar
    - Basil (dried)
    - Garlic (minced)
- One lemon (juiced)
- One tsp. of each
    - Salt
    - Oregano
- One pound of chicken thighs

For the salad:

- Four cups of lettuce leaves (washed)
- One cucumber (diced)
- Two tomatoes (diced)
- One onion (sliced)
- One avocado (sliced)
- One-third cup of kalamata olives (sliced)
- Wedges of lemon (for serving)

Method:

1. Whisk all the marinade ingredients in a bowl. Pour half of the marinade in a shallow dish. Store the remaining marinade for the dressing.

2. Add the pieces of chicken in the marinade dish and marinate for half an hour.

3. Mix all the ingredients for the salad in a mixing bowl and keep aside.

4. Heat some oil in a grill pan. Add the marinated chicken and cook for five minutes on each side until browned on all sides.

5. Slice the chicken pieces.

6. Serve the salad with chicken from the top. Drizzle some of the marinade and serve with lemon wedges.

Garlic Butter Scallops and Steak

Total Prep & Cooking Time: Thirty minutes

Yields: Two servings

Nutrition Facts: Calories: 280 | Protein: 23.1g | Carbs: 1.2g | Fat: 1.3g | Fiber: 0.3g

Ingredients

- Two fillets of beef tenderloin
- Black pepper and kosher salt (according to taste)
- Three tbsps. of butter
- Ten sea scallops

For the sauce:

- Three garlic cloves (minced)
- Six tbsps. of butter (cubed)
- Two tbsps. of each
    - Chives (chopped)
    - Parsley (chopped)
- One tbsp. of lemon juice
- Two tsps. of lemon zest
- Black pepper and kosher salt (according to taste)

Method:

1. Take an iron skillet and heat it over medium flame for ten minutes.
2. Season the steak with pepper and salt.

3. Add two tbsps. of butter in the skillet. Add the steak and cook for six minutes on each side. Cook until the steak reaches your desired doneness.

4. Keep the steak aside and heat one tbsp. of butter in the skillet.

5. Remove the muscles from the small side of the scallops and wash them with cold running water.

6. Season the scallops with pepper and salt. Cook the scallops on each side for three minutes.

7. For making the sauce, add garlic and butter in a skillet. Stir for one minute. Add chives, lemon zest, parsley, and lemon juice. Add pepper and salt for seasoning.

8. Serve the scallops and steak with butter sauce from the top.

Fried Chicken

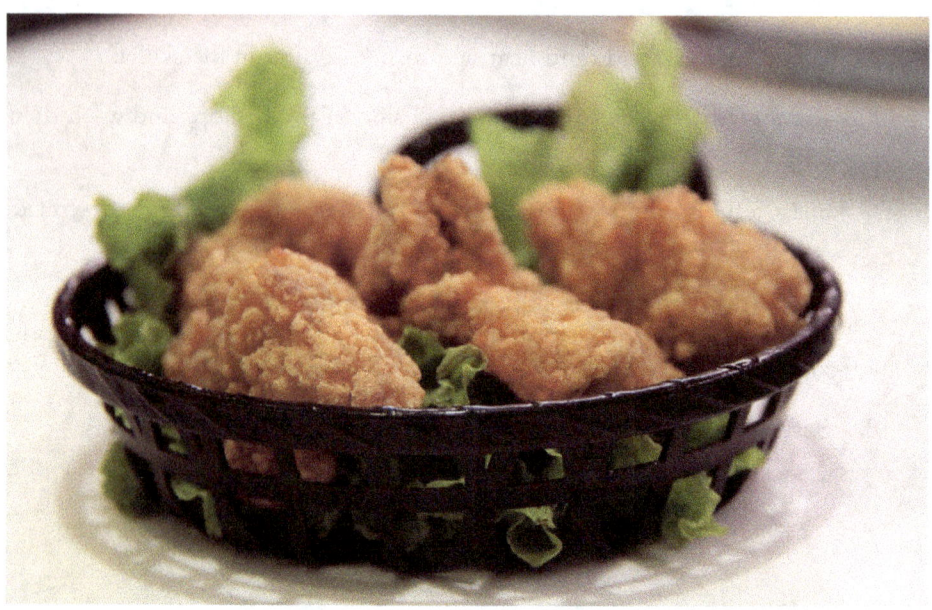

Total Prep & Cooking Time: Fifty minutes

Yields: Twelve servings

Nutrition Facts: Calories: 305 | Protein: 38.2g | Carbs: 0.6g | Fat: 12.3g | Fiber: 0.5g

Ingredients

- Four ounces of pork rinds
- Two tsps. of thyme (dried)
- One tsp. of each
    - Black pepper
    - Salt
    - Oregano (dried)
- Half tsp. of garlic powder

- One-third tsp. of paprika (smoked)
- Twelve chicken legs
- One large egg
- Two ounces of mayonnaise
- Three tbsps. of Dijon mustard

Method:

1. Crush the pork rinds for making powder texture. Leave some of the big pieces.

2. Preheat the oven at 200 degrees Celsius.

3. Mix salt, pork rinds, thyme, pepper, garlic powder, oregano, and paprika. Spread out the prepared mixture on a large flat dish.

4. Combine Dijon mustard, egg, and mayonnaise in a bowl. Dip the chicken legs in the egg mixture and then roll in the mixture of pork rind. Coat well.

5. Place the legs of chicken on a baking tray. Bake for forty minutes.

6. Serve hot.

Lime Chile Steak Fajitas

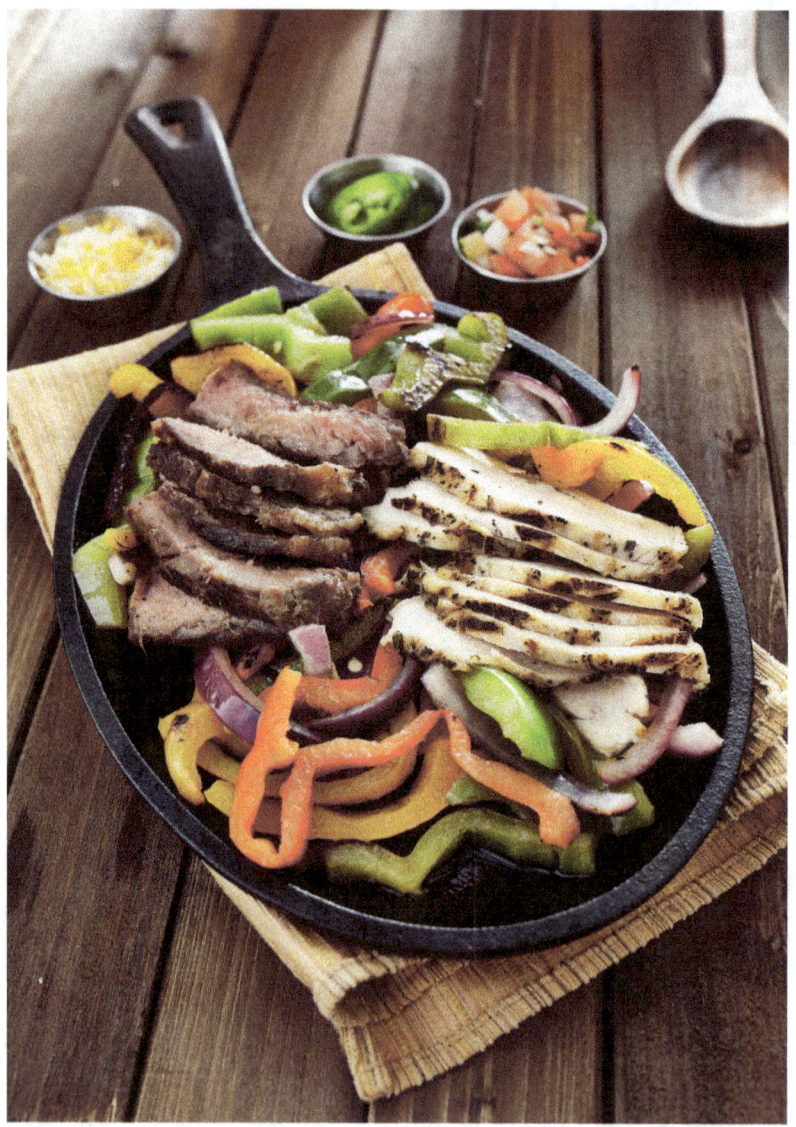

Total Prep & Cooking Time: Twenty-five minutes

Yields: Four servings

Nutrition Facts: Calories: 419 | Protein: 23.1g | Carbs: 12g | Fat: 25.6g | Fiber: 5.1g

Ingredients

For the marinade:

- Two tbsps. of olive oil
- One-third cup of lime juice
- Three tbsps. of cilantro (chopped)
- Two garlic cloves (chopped)
- One tsp. of brown sugar
- Three-fourth tsp. of chili flakes
- Half tsp. of cumin (ground)
- One tsp. of salt
- One pound of steak

For the fajitas:

- Three capsicums (different colors, sliced)
- One avocado (sliced)
- One onion (sliced)

For serving:

- Tortillas
- Sour cream

Method:

1. Combine all the marinade ingredients in a bowl. Keep aside half of the marinade. Pour the remaining marinade in a flat dish and marinate the steak.

2. Heat one tsp. of oil in a skillet. Add the steak and grill for five minutes on each side. Allow the steak to cool down for five minutes.

3. Wipe the skillet and brush some oil. Fry the capsicums along with the strips of onion. Add the reserved marinade, pepper, and salt.

4. For serving the steak, slice the steak. Arrange steak, sour cream, avocado, and cooked veggies in the tortillas. Serve with marinade and cilantro from the top.

Spaghetti Squash With Stuffed Lasagna

Total Prep & Cooking Time: Two hours

Yields: Four servings

Nutrition Facts: Calories: 280 | Protein: 23.1g | Carbs: 6.7g | Fat: 21.3g | Fiber: 0.2g

Ingredients

- One pound of Italian sausage
- One spaghetti squash
- One cup of pasta sauce (low-carb)
- One-fourth cup of ricotta
- One-third cup of mozzarella
- Half cup of parmesan
- Pepper and salt (according to taste)
- Parsley (for garnishing)

Method:

1. Cut spaghetti squash in half. Remove the seeds. Bake the squash in the oven with the cut side down in one inch of water. Bake for fifty minutes at 200 degrees Celsius.
2. Take a skillet and add the sausage. Cook until browned and add pasta sauce. Simmer for ten minutes and add seasonings.
3. Take out the baked squash and scrape the inside portion with the help of a fork. Add the squash strands in a bowl.
4. Combine the strands with ricotta, meat sauce, and cheese.
5. Stuff the squash shells with the mixture and arrange in a baking sheet. Top with mozzarella.
6. Bake the squash for fifteen minutes until the cheese melts.
7. Serve with parsley from the top.

Zucchini Boats With Stuffed Tuna

Total Prep & Cooking Time: Thirty minutes

Yields: Two servings

Nutrition Facts: Calories: 412 | Protein: 37.2g | Carbs: 23.2g | Fat: 18.3g | Fiber: 10.6g

Ingredients

- Two tsps. of avocado oil
- Half red bell pepper (diced)
- Two cans of wild tuna
- Half cup of salsa
- Two zucchinis
- Pepper and salt
- Half tsp. of cumin

For salsa

- One avocado (cubed)
- One-fourth cup of cilantro (chopped)
- Three tbsps. of onion (minced)
- Two tsps. of lime juice

Method:

1. Take a frying pan and heat oil in it. Add diced pepper and sauté for two minutes. Remove the pepper and add tuna. Cook for four minutes.
2. Add salsa to the pan. Combine well.
3. Trim the zucchini ends. Slice them in half, lengthwise. Use a spoon for scraping out the flesh. Sprinkle some cumin, pepper, and salt.
4. Fill the zucchini shells with tuna mixture.
5. Preheat your oven at 200 degrees Celsius.
6. Bake the zucchini for twenty minutes.
7. Mix the ingredients for the salsa in a large small mixing bowl.
8. Serve the zucchini boats with salsa by the side.

Spinach and Goat Cheese Stuffed Breast of Chicken

Total Prep & Cooking Time: Forty-five minutes

Yields: Four servings

Nutrition Facts: Calories: 229 | Protein: 27.8g | Carbs: 4.9g | Fat: 13.7g | Fiber: 2.8g

Ingredients

- Four breasts of chicken
- Two tbsps. of olive oil
- Four cups of spinach
- Half tsp. of garlic powder
- Two ounces of goat cheese
- One onion (sliced)
- Eight ounces of bella mushrooms
- One tsp. of thyme
- Pepper and salt (for seasoning)

Method:

1. Heat the oven at 175 degrees Celsius.
2. Use a sharp knife for cutting slits on the upper side of the chicken breasts. Drizzle the breasts with olive oil, pepper, and salt. Keep aside.
3. Take a large skillet and heat half tbsp. of oil in it. Add spinach and cook for two minutes. Add garlic powder and cook until the spinach wilts.
4. Transfer spinach to a bowl. Add the goat cheese. Combine well.
5. Stuff the slits of the chicken breasts with the cheese and spinach mixture.
6. Heat one tbsp. of oil in the same skillet. Add mushrooms, onion, and thyme. Season with pepper and salt. Cook until the onions caramelize. Move the cooked veggies to a side to make some room for the chicken breasts.
7. Add the stuffed chicken breasts to the skillet.
8. Put the skillet in the oven. Bake for thirty minutes.
9. Serve hot.

Chapter 2: Quick and Easy Recipes

When you are short of time, opting for quick and easy recipes is the best option. So, I have included some easy recipes in this section that you can make without any hassle.

Antipasto Salad

Total Prep & Cooking Time: Thirty minutes

Yields: Two servings

Nutrition Facts: Calories: 510 | Protein: 36.8g | Carbs: 12.4g | Fat: 61g | Fiber: 10.6g

Ingredients

- Ten ounces of lettuce (chopped in pieces)
- Two tbsps. of parsley (chopped)
- Five ounces of mozzarella cheese (sliced)
- Three ounces of each
    - Salami (sliced thinly)
    - Prosciutto (sliced thinly)
- Four ounces of canned artichokes (quartered)
- Two cups of roasted red pepper
- One ounce of each
    - Sun-dried tomatoes (chopped)
    - Olives (sliced)
- One-third cup of basil
- One chili pepper (chopped)
- Half tbsp. of salt
- Four tbsps. of olive oil

Method:

1. Distribute the leaves of lettuce on serving plates or on a large dish.

2. Add parsley from the top.

3. Layer all the ingredients of antipasto.

4. In a bowl, mix chopped chili, basil, and salt. Crush the ingredients using a wooden spoon.

5. Sprinkle the crushed mixture over the salad and serve with olive oil from the top.

Feta Cheese and Chicken Plate

Total Prep & Cooking Time: Ten minutes

Yields: Two servings

Nutrition Facts: Calories: 810 | Protein: 63.3g | Carbs: 8.7g | Fat: 71g | Fiber: 3.2g

Ingredients

- Five-hundred grams of rotisserie chicken
- Two cups of feta cheese
- Two tomatoes
- Three cups of lettuce
- Ten olives
- One-third cup of olive oil
- Pepper and salt (according to taste)

Method:

1. Arrange chicken, lettuce, cheese, and olives on a plate. Slice the tomatoes and arrange them on the plate.

2. Sprinkle pepper and salt for seasoning.

3. Serve with olive oil from the top.

Note: If you do not want to use rotisserie chicken, you can cook the chicken from scratch.

Cheese Omelet

Total Prep & Cooking Time: Fifteen minutes

Yields: Two servings

Nutrition Facts: Calories: 797 | Protein: 37.2g | Carbs: 3.9g | Fat: 74.2g | Fiber: 0.1g

Ingredients

- Half cup of butter
- Six large eggs
- One cup of cheddar cheese (shredded)
- Pepper and salt (according to taste)

Method:

1. Break the eggs in a bowl. Add the cheese and whisk. Season with pepper and salt.

2. Take a medium-sized pan and melt some butter in it. Add the whisked egg mixture and allow it to set for two minutes.

3. Reduce the flame and cook for four minutes on each side. Add the leftover cheese.

4. Fold the omelet in half. Cook for one more minute.

5. Serve hot.

Baked Salmon and Pesto

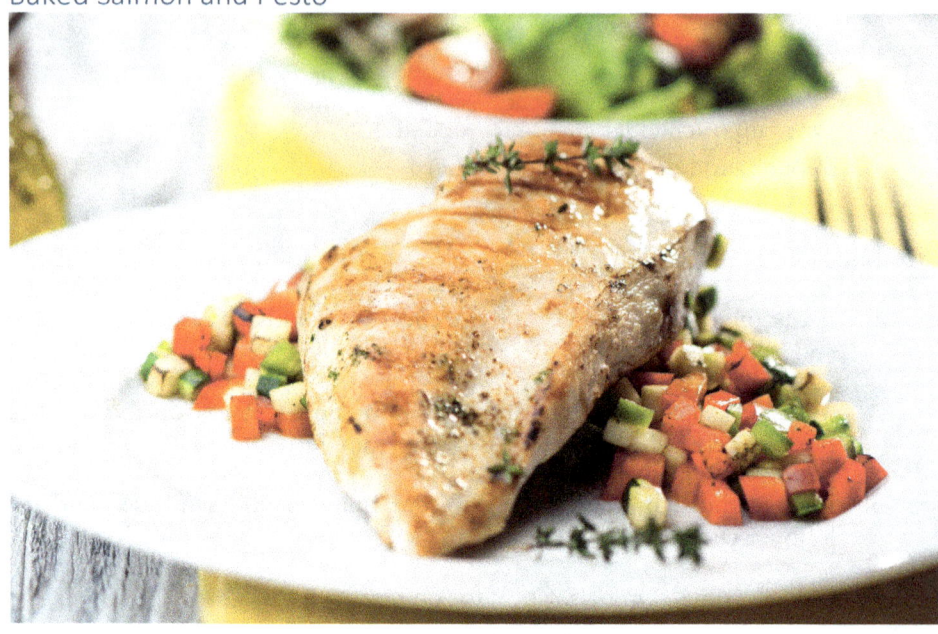

Total Prep & Cooking Time: Thirty minutes

Yields: Four servings

Nutrition Facts: Calories: 625 | Protein: 48.3g | Carbs: 3.2g | Fat: 89g | Fiber: 0.7g

Ingredients

- Four tbsps. of pesto
- One cup of mayonnaise
- Half cup of Greek yogurt
- Pepper and salt (according to taste)

For the salmon:

- Four fillets of salmon

- Four tbsps. of green pesto
- Pepper and salt (for seasoning)

Method:

1. Grease a baking dish with some oil. Place the fillets of salmon on the dish with the skin-side down. Spread green pesto on the fillets and season with pepper and salt.

2. Bake the salmon for thirty minutes at 200 degrees Celsius.

3. Stir the ingredients for the sauce in a bowl.

4. Serve the salmon with sauce from the top.

Pork Chops and Blue Cheese Sauce

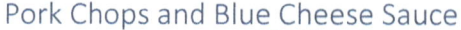

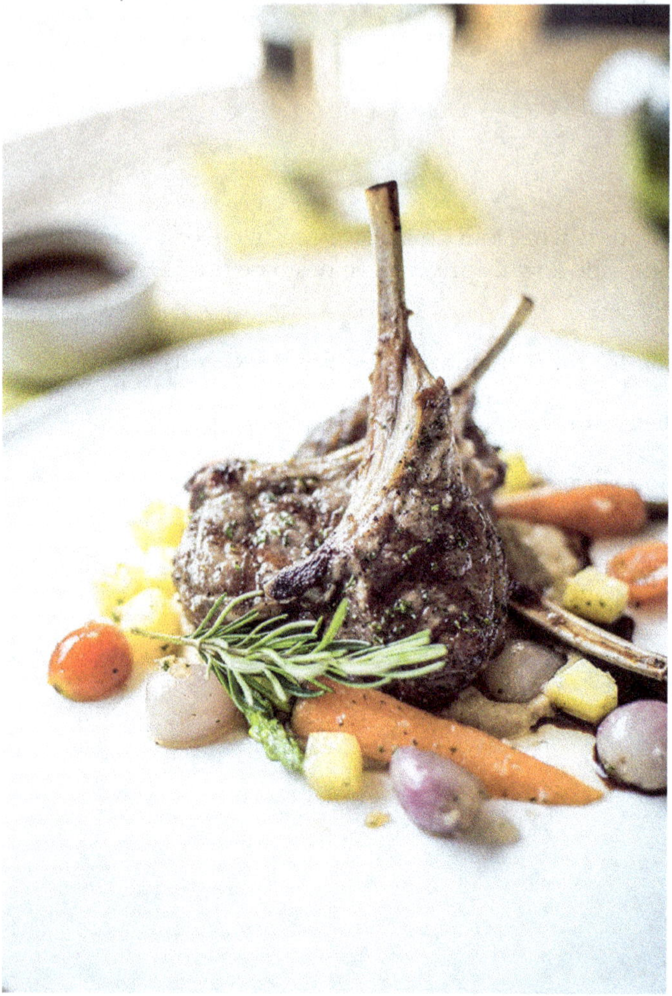

Total Prep & Cooking Time: Twenty minutes

Yields: Four servings

Nutrition Facts: Calories: 669 | Protein: 53.2g | Carbs: 4.3g | Fat: 60.1g | Fiber: 1.6g

Ingredients

- Two cups of blue cheese
- One cup of whipping cream (heavy)
- Four pork chops
- Seven ounces of green beans
- Two tbsps. of butter
- Pepper and salt

Method:

1. Crumble the blue cheese in a pot. Place the pot over medium flame and allow the cheese to melt.

2. Add whipping cream in the melted cheese and mix well. Simmer for two minutes.

3. Season the chops using pepper and salt.

4. Take an iron skillet and heat some oil in it. Add the chops and cook for four minutes on each side.

5. Add the juices from the pan in the sauce and stir.

6. Trim the beans. Heat some oil butter in the skillet and sauté the beans for two minutes.

7. Serve the pork chops with cheese sauce from the top and beans by the side.

Green Pepper and Pork Stir-Fry

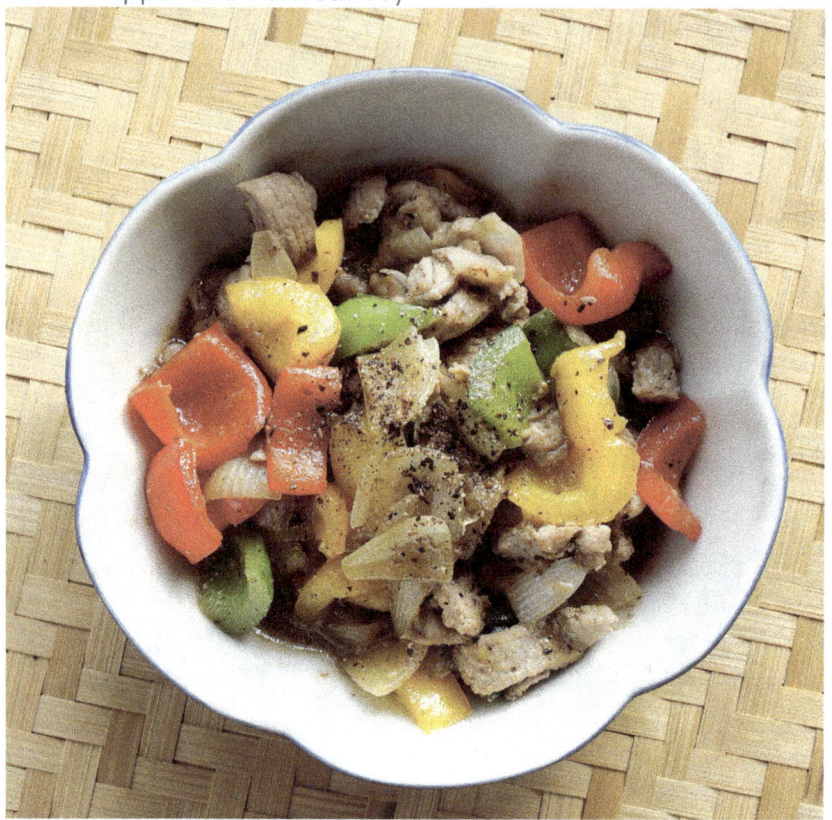

Total Prep & Cooking Time: Twenty-five minutes

Yields: Two servings

Nutrition Facts: Calories: 678 | Protein: 31.2g | Carbs: 5.3g | Fat: 71.3g | Fiber: 4.6g

Ingredients

- Four ounces of butter
- Four-hundred grams of pork shoulder (cut in strips)
- Two bell pepper (green, sliced)
- Two scallions (sliced)
- Half cup of almond
- One tsp. of chili paste
- Pepper and salt

Method:

1. Heat butter in a wok. Add the meat strips in the butter and cook for five minutes until browned.

2. Add the chili paste along with veggies. Cook for two minutes. Add pepper and salt.

3. Serve the stir-fry with almonds from the top.

Broccoli With Fried Chicken

Total Prep & Cooking Time: Thirty minutes

Yields: Two servings

Nutrition Facts: Calories: 633 | Protein: 30.1g | Carbs: 5.3g | Fat: 64.3g | Fiber: 3.6g

Ingredients

- Nine ounces of broccoli
- One cup of butter
- Ten ounces of chicken thighs (boneless)
- Pepper and salt
- Half cup of mayonnaise

Method:

1. Rinse the broccoli thoroughly under running water. Trim the florets along with the stem.

2. Heat some butter in a pan.

3. Season the chicken thighs. Add the chicken to the pan and cook them for five minutes on all sides.

4. Add some more butter in the pan and add the broccoli. Toss the broccoli and chicken and cook for two minutes.

5. Serve with mayonnaise from the top.

Fried Eggs With Pork and Kale
Total Prep & Cooking Time: Twenty-five minutes

Yields: Three servings

Nutrition Facts: Calories: 910 | Protein: 24g | Carbs: 7.6g | Fat: 89g | Fiber: 6.3g

Ingredients

- One cup of kale
- Three ounces of butter
- Six ounces of bacon or pork belly (smoked)
- One ounce of walnuts
- Four large eggs
- Pepper and salt

Method:

1. Chop the kale and wash them under cold water.
2. Melt some butter in a skillet and cook the kale for two minutes until the edges are slightly browned.
3. Remove kale from the skillet and keep aside. Add bacon or pork belly in the same skillet and sear until crispy.
4. Add the kale in the skillet along with walnuts. Toss the ingredients.
5. Heat butter in another pan and fry the eggs sunny side up. Add pepper and salt for seasoning.
6. Serve the eggs with kale mixture by the side.

Chapter 3: Sweet Recipes

Even when you are on a diet, you don't have to compromise on satisfying your sweet tooth. So, I have included some easy to make sweet keto recipes in this section.

Sugar Cinnamon Donuts

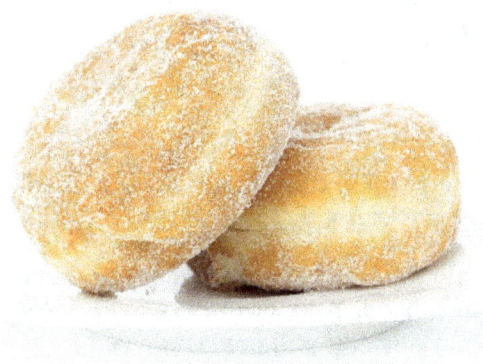

Total Prep & Cooking Time: Twenty-five minutes

Yields: Twelve servings

Nutrition Facts: Calories: 82 | Protein: 2.3g | Carbs: 1.9g | Fat: 7.8g | Fiber: 0.3g

Ingredients

- Two eggs
- One-fourth cup of almond milk
- One-fourth tsp. of apple cider vinegar
- One tsp. of vanilla extract
- Two tbsps. of butter
- One-third cup of sweetener
- One cup of fine almond flour
- Half tbsp. of coconut flour
- One tsp. of cinnamon (ground)
- One and a half tsp. of baking powder
- Half tsp. of baking soda
- Half cup of salt

For sugar cinnamon coating:

- One-fourth cup of granulated erythritol
- One tsp. of cinnamon (ground)
- Two tbsps. of butter

Method:

1. Whisk together almond milk, eggs, butter, vinegar, vanilla extract, and sweetener. Combine until smooth.

2. Combine coconut flour, almond flour, baking powder, cinnamon, salt, and baking soda in a bowl. Add all the dry ingredients slowly to the mixture of wet ingredients. Stir well until combined.

3. Transfer the donut batter into a donut pan.

4. Bake the donuts for fifteen minutes at 175 degrees Celsius.

5. Take out the donuts and keep aside for cooling.

6. Stir together cinnamon and sweetener in a bowl.

7. Melt the butter in a pan.

8. Take the donuts and dunk them in the butter. Roll the donuts in the cinnamon coating.

Mug Brownie

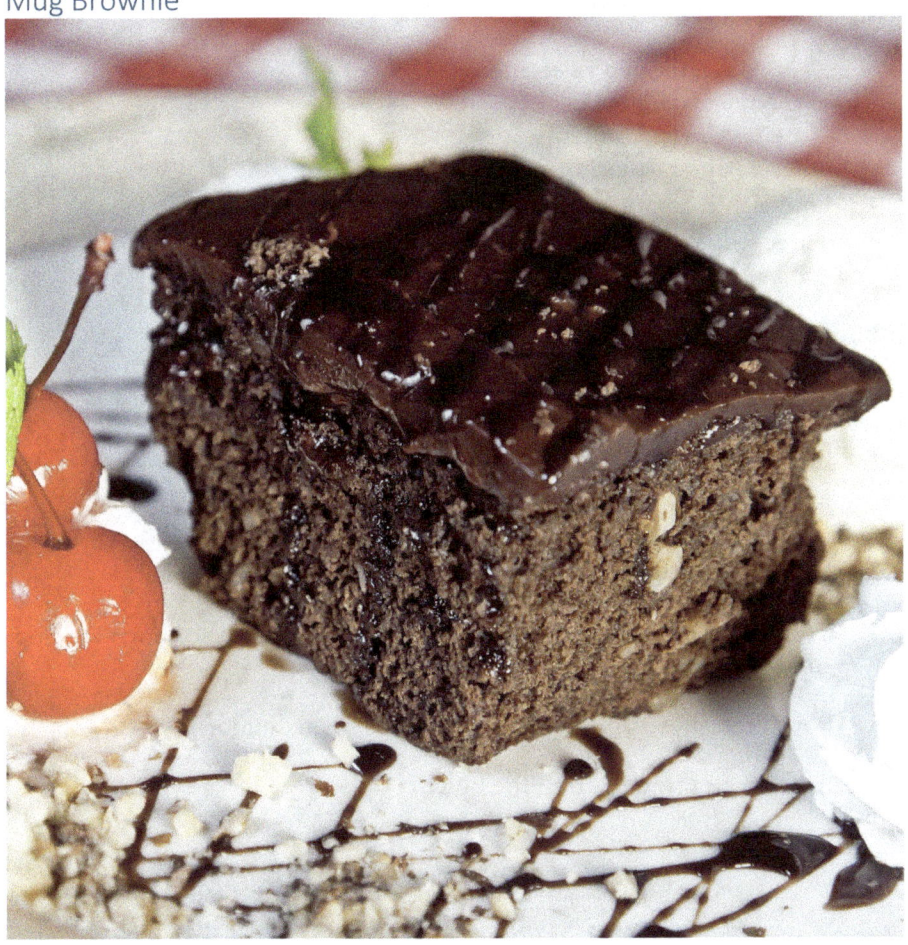

Total Prep & Cooking Time: Ten minutes

Yields: Two servings

Nutrition Facts: Calories: 194 | Protein: 7.9g | Carbs: 7.6g | Fat: 16.5g | Fiber: 6.7g

Ingredients

- Two tbsps. of almond flour
- One tbsp. of each
    - Granulated sweetener
    - Cocoa powder
    - Almond butter
    - Chocolate chips
- One-eighth tsp. of baking powder
- Three tbsps. of milk

Method:

1. Use a cooking spray for greasing cereal bowls or mugs.
2. Combine the listed dry ingredients. Mix properly.
3. Mix milk and almond butter in a separate bowl and mix well.
4. Combine the dry and wet ingredients. Mix well. Add the chocolate chips and fold well.
5. Pour the batter in the cereal bowls. Bake for six minutes.
6. Enjoy your brownie from the bowl.

Mini Cheesecake

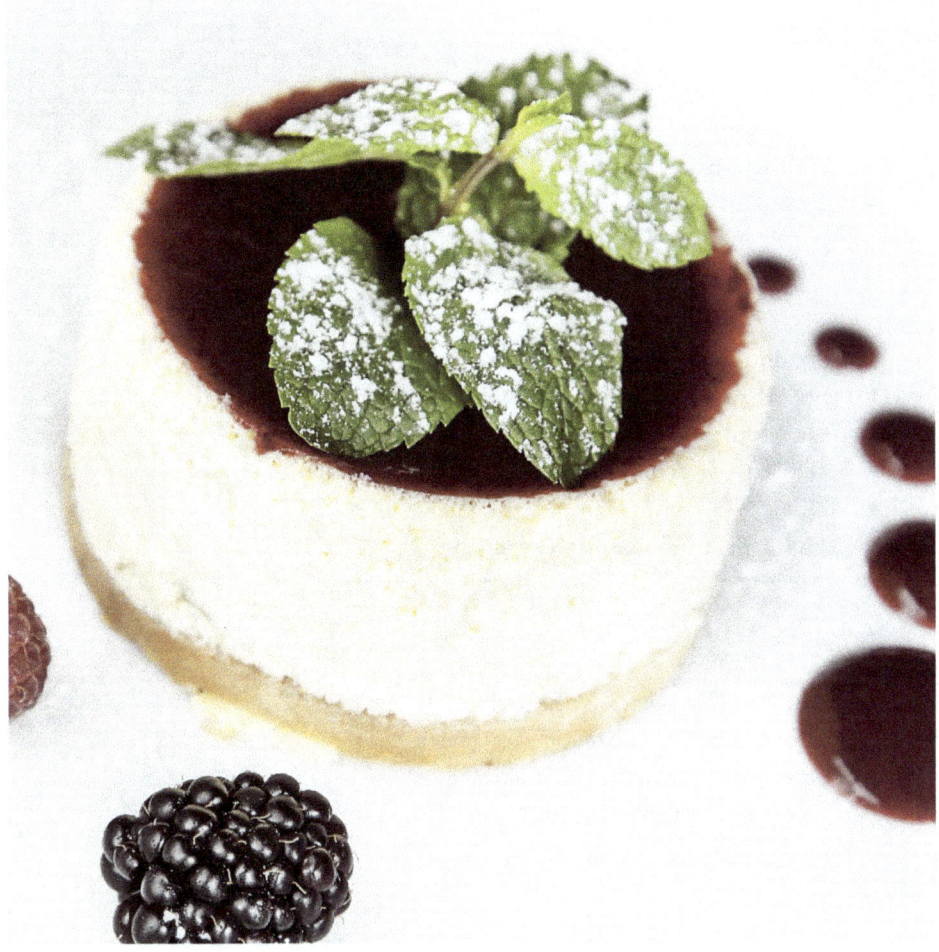

Total Prep & Cooking Time: Three hours and twenty minutes

Yields: Six servings

Nutrition Facts: Calories: 230 | Protein: 4.7g | Carbs: 5.1g | Fat: 19.6g | Fiber: 1.8g

Ingredients

For the crust:

- Half cup of almond flour
- Two tbsps. of sweetener
- Half tsp. of cinnamon
- Two tbsps. of butter (melted)

For the filling:

- Six ounces of cream cheese (softened)
- Five tbsps. of sweetener
- One-fourth cup of sour cream
- Half tsp. of vanilla extract
- One egg
- Two tsps. of cinnamon (ground)

For the frosting:

- One tbsp. of butter (softened)
- Three tbsps. of confectioners sweetener
- One-fourth tsp. of vanilla extract
- Two tsps. of heavy cream

Method:

1. Heat the oven at 175 degrees Celsius. Line a small muffin pan with six silicone liners.

2. Whisk almond flour, cinnamon, and sweetener in a bowl. Add melted butter and mix well.

3. Divide the prepared crust among the muffin cups. Press the crust to the bottom. Bake in the oven for five minutes.

4. Beat three tbsps. of sweetener along with the cream cheese in a bowl. Add vanilla, egg, and sour cream. Beat well.

5. Reduce oven temperature to 160 degrees Celsius.

6. Whisk cinnamon and butter in a bowl.

7. Add three-fourth tbsp. of cheese mixture into the muffin cups. Sprinkle cinnamon mixture from the top.

8. Bake the muffins for fifteen minutes. Refrigerate the muffins for two hours.

9. Beat powdered sweetener and butter in a bowl. Add heavy cream and vanilla extract. Mix well.

10. Transfer the frosting to a zip-lock bag and cut a small hole at the corner.

11. Add frosting over the cheesecakes.

Keto Fudge

Total Prep & Cooking Time: One hour

Yields: Twelve servings

Nutrition Facts: Calories: 158 | Protein: 0.1g | Carbs: 0.6g | Fat: 17.9g | Fiber: 0.7g

Ingredients

- One cup of coconut oil
- One-fourth cup of each
    - Cocoa powder
    - Erythritol (powdered)
- One tsp. of vanilla extract
- One-eighth tsp. of sea salt
- Sea salt

Method:

1. Use parchment paper for lining a glass baking dish.
2. Beat sweetener and coconut oil using a hand blender. Make sure the mixture is fluffy.
3. Add vanilla extract, cocoa powder, and salt. Combine well.
4. Pour the fudge mixture in the lined dish. Smoothen the top using a spoon or spatula.
5. Refrigerate the fudge for forty minutes until it solidifies.
6. Use a sharp knife to run along the edges of the dish for taking out the fudge.
7. Cut in small cubes and serve.

Peanut Butter Hearts

Total Prep & Cooking Time: Thirty minutes

Yields: Twenty servings

Nutrition Facts: Calories: 91 | Protein: 5.1g | Carbs: 7.1g | Fat: 6.7g | Fiber: 5.2g

Ingredients

- Two cups of peanut butter
- Three-fourth cup of any sticky sweetener
- One cup of coconut flour
- One and a half cup of chocolate chips

Method:

1. Use parchment paper for lining a large glass tray.
2. Combine sticky sweetener with peanut butter on the stovetop. Combine the mixture until it melts completely.
3. Add the coconut flour and combine. In case the batter is very thin, you can add more flour.
4. Make twenty balls from the dough. Use a heart-shaped cookie cutter for pressing the dough balls for making heart shape.
5. Arrange the hearts on the lined glass tray and refrigerate.
6. Melt the chocolate chips and dip the hearts in the melted chocolate.
7. Refrigerate again for twenty minutes until firm.

Peanut Butter and White Chocolate Blondies

Total Prep & Cooking Time: Three hours and thirty-five minutes

Yields: Sixteen servings

Nutrition Facts: Calories: 102 | Protein: 3.2g | Carbs: 2.2g | Fat: 9.3g | Fiber: 1.9g

Ingredients

- Half cup of each
    - Peanut butter
    - Sweetener of your choice
- Four tbsps. of butter (softened)
- Two large eggs
- One tsp. of vanilla extract
- Three tbsps. of cocoa butter (melted)
- One-fourth cup of almond flour
- One tbsp. of coconut flour
- One cup of cocoa butter (chopped)

Method:

1. Heat the oven at 175 degrees Celsius. Use a cooking spray for greasing a baking dish.
2. Combine all the ingredients in a large bowl using a hand mixer.
3. Pour the mixture in the greased dish.
4. Bake for thirty minutes.
5. Cool the blondies and refrigerate for about three hours.
6. Cut the blondies in squares and serve.

Low Carb Ice Cream

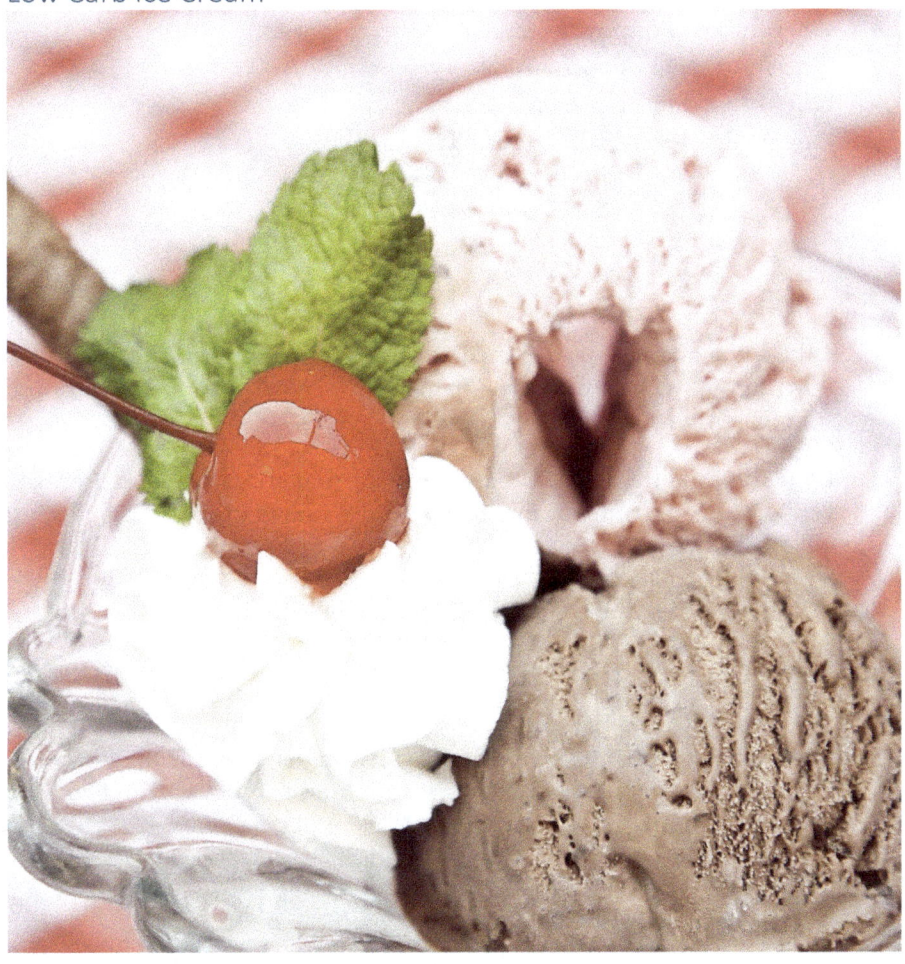

Total Prep & Cooking Time: Five hours and thirty-five minutes

Yields: Eight servings

Nutrition Facts: Calories: 337 | Protein: 2.2g | Carbs: 3.1g | Fat: 34g | Fiber: 0.3g

Ingredients

- Three tbsps. of butter

- Three cups of heavy cream
- One-third cup of powdered allulose
- One-fourth cup of coconut oil
- One tsp. of vanilla extract
- One medium-sized bean of vanilla

Method:

1. Take a pan and heat it over medium flame. Melt butter in it. Add a two-third cup of the heavy cream along with sweetener. Boil the mixture and simmer for thirty minutes.

2. Pour the mixture in a bowl and let it cool at room temperature. Add vanilla seeds from the bean along with the vanilla extract. Add coconut oil and mix well.

3. Add the remaining cream and combine until smooth.

4. Pour the mixture in a container and use a spatula for smoothening the top.

5. Freeze the ice cream for five hours. Ensure that you stir the ice cream mixture after every thirty minutes for the first two hours and then after every sixty minutes.

Chocolate Donut

Total Prep & Cooking Time: One hour and twenty-five minutes

Yields: Ten servings

Nutrition Facts: Calories: 219 | Protein: 5.1g | Carbs: 7.6g | Fat: 18.6g | Fiber: 3.1g

Ingredients

- Four eggs
- Half cup of butter (melted)
- Three tbsps. of milk
- One tsp. of stevia
- One-fourth cup of each
    - Coconut flour
    - Cocoa powder (unsweetened)
    - Sea salt
    - Baking soda

For the glaze:

- One tbsp. of avocado oil
- Three-fourth cup of chocolate chips

Method:

1. Heat the oven at 175 degrees Celsius.
2. Use a cooking spray for greasing donut pan of ten cavities.
3. Mix melted butter, eggs, and stevia, and milk in a bowl.
4. Add cocoa powder, coconut flour, baking soda, and salt.
5. Pour the mixture in the donut pan. Bake the donuts for fifteen minutes until set.
6. Let the donuts cool for fifteen minutes.
7. Add the chocolate chips in a bowl and melt in the microwave. Add avocado oil and stir.
8. Take out the donuts and dip them in the chocolate glaze.
9. Let the donuts sit for thirty minutes.

Chapter 4: Savory Recipes

In this section, I have included some tasty savory keto recipes that you can enjoy at any time of the day. So, let's have a look at them.

Keto McMuffin

Total Prep & Cooking Time: Twenty minutes

Yields: Two servings

Nutrition Facts: Calories: 610 | Protein: 24g | Carbs: 3.2g | Fat: 51.8g | Fiber: 6.9g

Ingredients

- One-fourth cup of each
    - Almond flour
    - Flaxmeal
- One-fourth tsp. of baking soda
- One egg
- Two tbsps. of heavy whipping cream
- One cup of cheddar cheese (shredded)
- Three tbsps. of water
- Salt (for seasoning)

For the filling:

- Two large eggs
- One tbsp. of butter
- Two cheddar cheese slices
- One tsp. of Dijon mustard
- Pepper and salt (for seasoning)

Method:

1. Combine all the dry ingredients. Mix well.
2. Add cream, water, and egg. Combine well using a fork.
3. Add the shredded cheese and mix.
4. Pour the mixture in greased ramekins. Microwave the mixture at high settings for two minutes.
5. Take a pan and fry the eggs. Add pepper and salt for seasoning.
6. Cut the prepared muffins in half. Spread butter on the inside portion of the muffin halves.
7. Top the muffin slices with egg, cheese, and mustard.
8. Serve immediately.

Sausage Hash With Rainbow Chard

Total Prep & Cooking Time: Twenty-five minutes

Yields: Two servings

Nutrition Facts: Calories: 570 | Protein: 25g | Carbs: 7.6g | Fat: 44.6g | Fiber: 5.6g

Ingredients

- Two-hundred grams of Swiss chard
- Two cups of cauliflower rice
- One-hundred and fifty grams of sausage meat
- Three tbsps. of lard
- Two garlic cloves (chopped)
- One tbsp. of lemon juice
- One tsp. of Dijon mustard
- Pepper and salt
- Four poached eggs

Method:

1. Chop the chard stalks into small pieces.
2. Take a greased skillet and add the sausage meat. Cook for five minutes until browned. Keep aside
3. Add the remaining lard to the same skillet. Add the garlic. Cook for one minute and add the cauliflower rice. Cook the mixture for five minutes.
4. Add the chard and Dijon mustard. Combine well. Add lemon juice and cook the mixture for two minutes. Add pepper and salt for seasoning.
5. Add the sausage meat and mix.
6. Serve with poached eggs.

Veggie and Chicken Sausage Skillet
Total Prep & Cooking Time: Thirty minutes

Yields: Four servings

Nutrition Facts: Calories: 310 | Protein: 21g | Carbs: 9.3g | Fat: 22.3g | Fiber: 2.4g

Ingredients

- Three tbsps. of butter
- Five links of chicken sausage (sliced)
- Two garlic cloves (minced)
- One red onion (cut in chunks)
- One zucchini (sliced in rounds)
- One summer squash (sliced in rounds)
- One red capsicum (cut in chunks)
- One yellow capsicum (cut in chunks)
- Six cremini mushrooms (quartered)
- Half tsp. of each
    - Red pepper flakes (crushed)
    - Italian seasoning
- Pepper and salt

Method:

1. Take an iron skillet and melt some butter in it.
2. Add the sausage, onion, and garlic. Sauté the mixture for ten minutes.
3. Add the veggies and mix well. Add pepper flakes, Italian seasoning, pepper, and salt.
4. Sauté the mixture for fifteen minutes and serve hot.

Cheese and Crispy Salami

Total Prep & Cooking Time: Twenty-five minutes

Yields: Ten servings

Nutrition Facts: Calories: 37 | Protein: 2.3g | Carbs: 1.3g | Fat: 2.7g | Fiber: 6.3g

Ingredients

- Two ounces of dried salami
- One ounce of cream cheese
- Half cup of parsley (chopped)

Method:

1. Heat the oven at 170 degrees Celsius.
2. Slice the salami into thirty slices of a quarter inch.
3. Arrange the salami on a baking pan.
4. Bake them for fifteen minutes.
5. Top the salami with cream cheese along with parsley.

Buffalo Chicken Sandwich

Total Prep & Cooking Time: Twenty-five minutes

Yields: Four servings

Nutrition Facts: Calories: 480 | Protein: 27g | Carbs: 5.1g | Fat: 30g | Fiber: 2.2g

Ingredients

- Two cups of cooked chicken (shredded)
- One-third cup of red pepper sauce
- Three tbsps. of butter
- One-fourth tsp. of each
    - Celery seed spice
    - Sea salt
    - Garlic powder
- Two tbsps. of each
    - Blue cheese crumbles
    - Celery (minced)
- Four tbsps. of ranch dressing
- Three tbsps. of mayonnaise
- Four sandwich buns

Method

1. Take a medium saucepan and melt butter in it. Add celery seed spice, red pepper sauce, sea salt, and garlic powder. Stir well.
2. Add the chicken along with celery to the pan. Mix well and cook for two minutes.
3. Add the mayonnaise and combine.
4. Cut the buns in half. Add half cup of prepared chicken mixture on the buns. Top the chicken with one tbsp. of ranch dressing and half tbsp. of cheese crumbles.
5. Place the other halves on top and serve.

Cream Cheese and Salmon Bites
Total Prep & Cooking Time: Twenty minutes

Yields: Ten servings

Nutrition Facts: Calories: 43 | Protein: 1.3g | Carbs: 0.3g | Fat: 4.6g | Fiber: 0.6g

Ingredients

- Two eggs
- Half cup of cream
- One tbsp. of salt
- One cup of cheese (shredded)
- One-third tsp. of dill (dried)
- One-third cup of cream cheese (diced)
- Two cups of salmon (smoked, chopped)

Method:

1. Combine cream, eggs, and salt in a bowl.

2. Add cheese, cream cheese, and dill. Mix well.

3. Grease a muffin tray with butter.

4. Pour the mixture in the muffin tray. Add some pieces of salmon into each muffin.

5. Bake the mixture in the oven for twenty minutes at 180 degrees Celsius.

6. Remove the bites and serve warm. Vegetable Turkey Pesto Bolognese

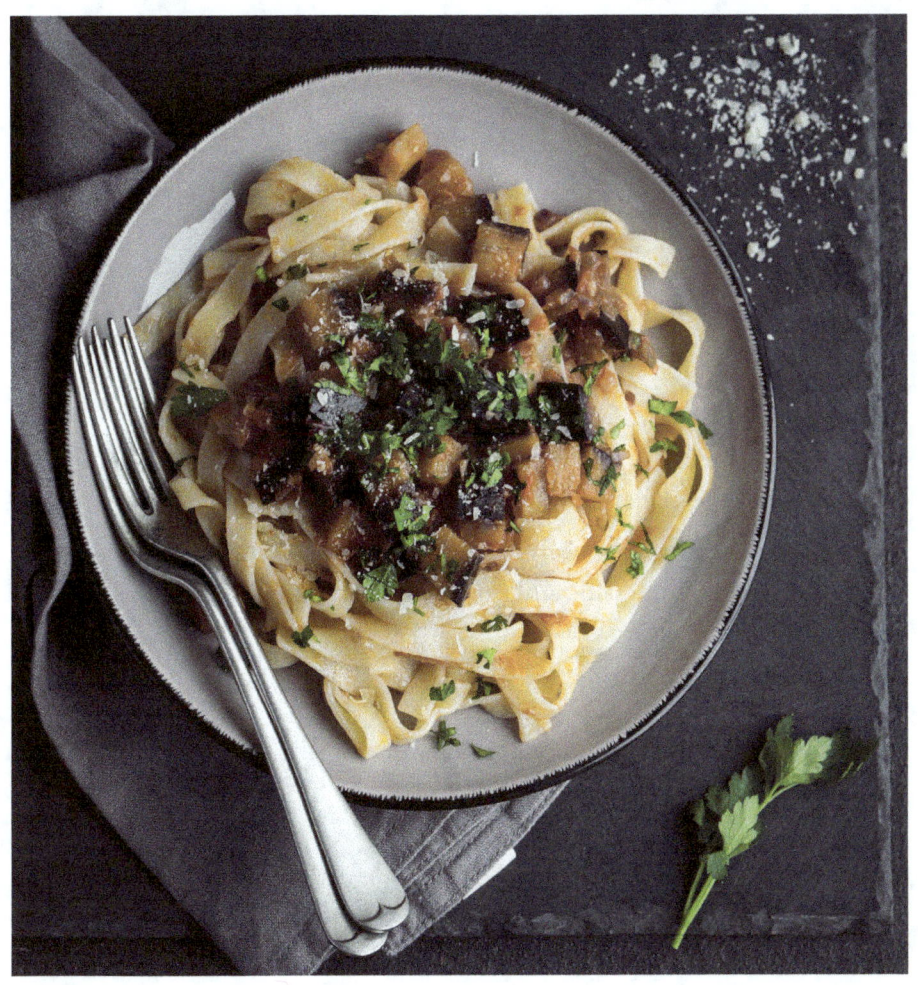

Total Prep & Cooking Time: Thirty minutes

Yields: Four servings

Nutrition Facts: Calories: 270 | Protein: 20.1g | Carbs: 4.3g | Fat: 13.2g | Fiber: 1.6g

Ingredients

- Two tsps. of oil

- One pound of turkey (ground)
- One cup of onion (diced)
- Two cups of each
    - Mushrooms (sliced)
    - Zucchini (sliced)
- Three tbsps. of pesto sauce
- Pasta of your choice (cooked)
- Grated cheese

Method:

1. Take a large skillet and add some oil. Add the turkey and cook until browned. Keep aside.

2. Add onions in the same and cook for two minutes. Add mushrooms and zucchini. Mix well.

3. Add the cooked turkey and combine it. Add pesto sauce simmer for five minutes.

4. Add cooked pasta along with cheese. Stir to combine. Simmer for two minutes.

5. Serve hot.

Turkey Patties

Total Prep & Cooking Time: Thirty minutes

Yields: Four servings

Nutrition Facts: Calories: 435 | Protein: 24g | Carbs: 4.5g | Fat: 37.2g | Fiber: 2.5g

Ingredients

- Five-hundred grams of ground turkey
- Half cup of almond flour
- One hot chili pepper (finely chopped)
- Two tsps. of Dijon mustard
- Two tbsps. of each
    - Parsley (chopped)
    - Lemon juice
    - Basil (chopped)
- Half tsp. of sea salt
- One tsp. black pepper (ground)
- Two spring onions (sliced finely)
- Two tbsps. of lard
- One egg
- Two garlic cloves (crushed)

Method:

1. Combine turkey, eggs, almond flour, garlic, pepper, lemon juice, Dijon mustard, basil, parsley, black pepper, and salt. Add the spring onions and mix well.

2. Make small patties using your hands.

3. Heat lard in a pan and add the patties. Cook the patties for five minutes on each side.

4. Let the patties sit for two minutes. Serve warm with spring onions.

Chapter 5: Poultry and Meat Recipes

Meat and poultry are rich in protein and various other nutrients that you need for perfect health. In this section, you will find some tasty poultry and meat keto recipes that you can make at home.

Beef Cabbage Skillet

Total Prep & Cooking Time: Thirty minutes

Yields: Four servings

Nutrition Facts: Calories: 357 | Protein: 13g | Carbs: 27g | Fat: 7.2g | Fiber: 11.3g

Ingredients

- Half green cabbage (shredded)
- Two tbsps. of butter
- One pound of beef (ground)
- Three tbsps. of taco seasoning
- One tsp. of minced onion (dried)
- One and a half cup of Mexican cheese blend
- Pepper and salt (according to taste)

Method:

1. Take a large skillet and heat one tbsp. of butter in it. Add shredded cabbage and sauté for two minutes. Keep aside.

2. Add one tbsp. of butter in the same skillet. Add the beef. Add onion, taco seasoning, and mix well. Cook for five minutes. Add one-fourth cup of water. Add the cooked cabbage along with pepper and salt. Combine half a cup of cheese.

3. Top with leftover cheese and place the skillet in the oven. Bake for ten minutes or until the cheese melts.

Meatball Casserole

Total Prep & Cooking Time: Three hours and thirty minutes

Yields: Six servings

Nutrition Facts: Calories: 470 | Protein: 37g | Carbs: 5.4g | Fat: 33.2g | Fiber: 4.7g

Ingredients

- Two pounds of beef (ground)
- Half cup of each
    - Mozzarella cheese
    - Parmesan cheese
- Two tbsps. of coconut flour
- Two large eggs
- Three-fourth tsp. of each
    - Onion (minced)
    - Salt
- One-fourth tsp. of Italian seasoning
- Half tsp. of garlic powder
- Twenty ounce can of spaghetti sauce
- Two cups of mozzarella cheese
- One tsp. of dried basil

Method:

1. Mix the ingredients in a bowl except for the spaghetti sauce, basil, and two cups of mozzarella cheese.
2. Heat a skillet on medium flame. Add one-fourth inch of coconut oil in the skillet.
3. Scoop meatballs from the mixture and add them to the skillet.

4. Cook the meatballs for five minutes until browned.//
5. Place the meatballs in the base of a crockpot.
6. Add spaghetti sauce from the top.
7. Cook the meatballs on high for three hours.
8. Take out the meatballs in a baking dish.
9. Sprinkle cheese from the top.
10. Broil the meatballs for three minutes until cheese melts.

Beef Taquitos
Total Prep & Cooking Time: Forty minutes

Yields: Six servings

Nutrition Facts: Calories: 229 | Protein: 15.7g | Carbs: 1.6g | Fat: 16.3g | Fiber: 0.3g

Ingredients

- One cup of each
    - Cheddar cheese (shredded)
    - Mozzarella cheese (shredded)
- Half cup of parmesan cheese (grated)
- Half pound of beef (ground)
- One-fourth cup of onion (minced)
- Half tsp. of each
    - Paprika
    - Chili powder
    - Salt
    - Onion powder
    - Garlic powder
- One tsp. of cumin
- One-fourth tsp. of pepper
- One-third cup of water

Method:

1. Mix chili powder, cumin, garlic powder, onion powder, pepper, salt in a cup, and some water.

2. Take a skillet and brown the beef along with the onion. Add the mixture over the beef and simmer for ten minutes.

3. Mix all the cheese in a bowl. Divide the mixture of cheese for making six balls. Use parchment paper to line a baking sheet. Place them on the sheet and bake for eight minutes.

4. Let the cheese sheets cool down for two minutes.

5. Take one spoon of the beef mixture and place it on the edge of the cheese sheets. Repeat for the remaining sheets.

6. Roll them tightly for making cigar shape.

7. Serve warm.

Chicken Wings

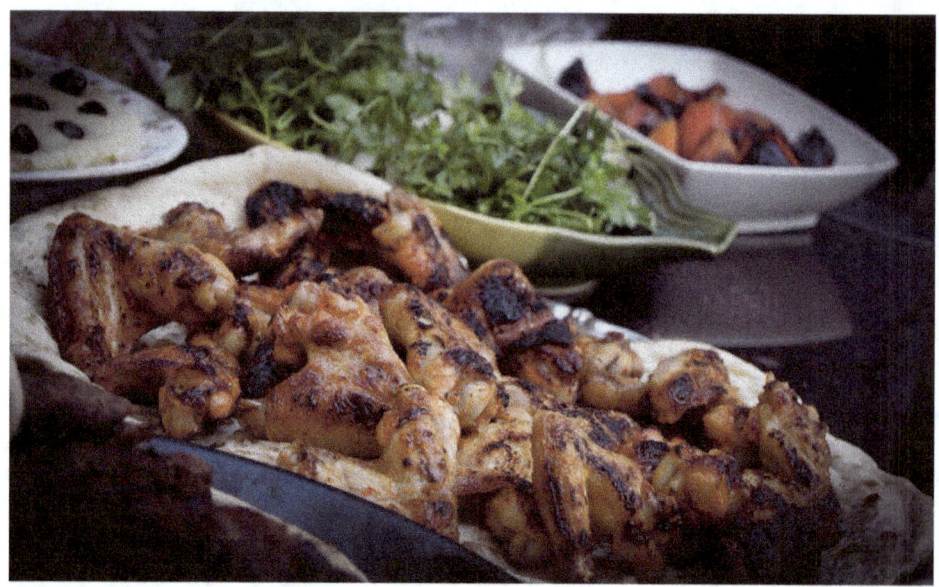

Total Prep & Cooking Time: Fifty minutes

Yields: Four servings

Nutrition Facts: Calories: 287 | Protein: 2.3g | Carbs: 12g | Fat: 16.3g | Fiber: 1.9g

Ingredients

- Two pounds of chicken wings
- Two tsps. of salt
- Three-fourth cup of coconut aminos
- One-fourth tsp. of each
    - Onion powder
    - Ginger (ground)
    - Garlic powder
    - Chili flakes

Method:

1. Place the wings on a baking tray.

2. Sprinkle some salt evenly on the wings.

3. Bake the chicken wings in the oven for forty minutes at 180 degrees Celsius.

4. Take a skillet and add coconut aminos. Add garlic powder, ginger, onion powder, and chili flakes. Simmer the sauce and stir until the sauce thickens.

5. Place the cooked wings in a large bowl and pour the sauce over the wings. Toss the cooked wings in the prepared sauce. Coat evenly.

6. Serve hot.

Roasted Leg of Chicken

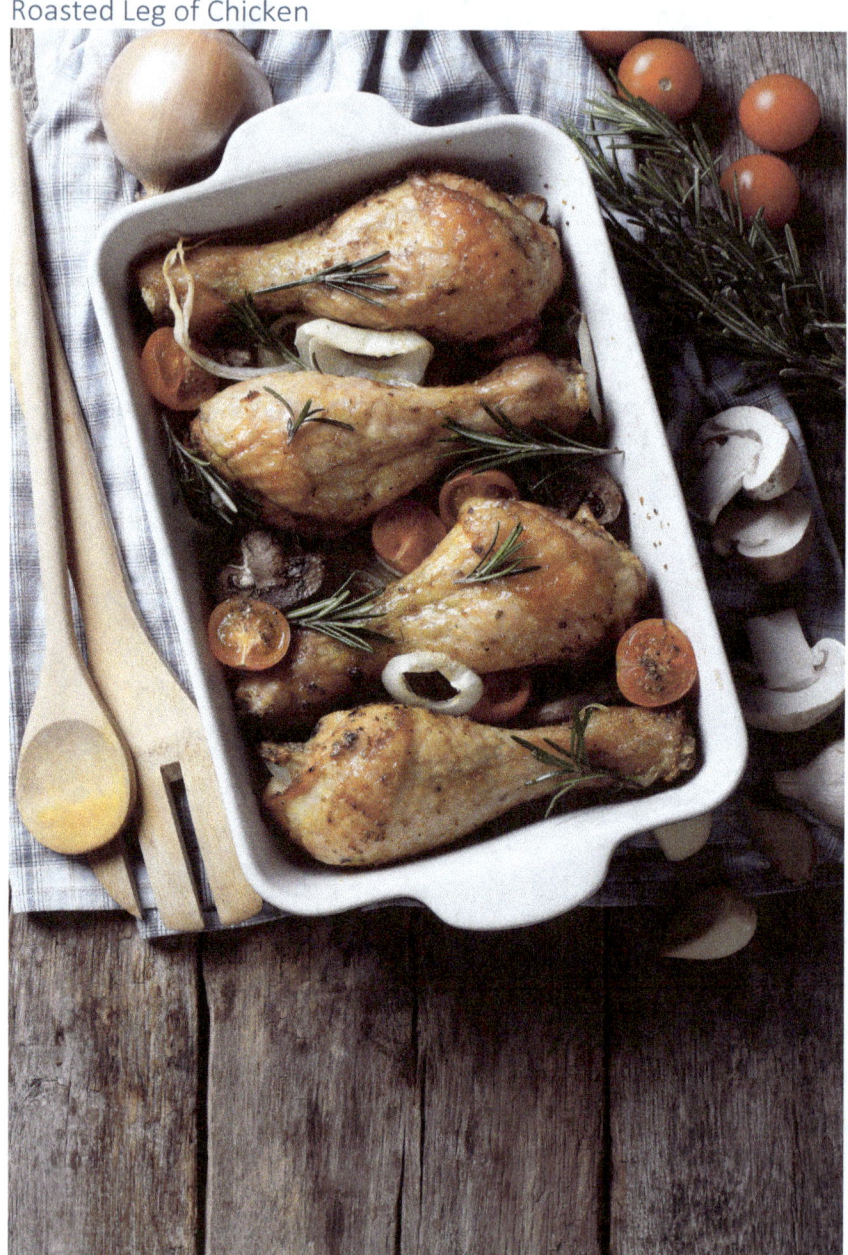

Total Prep & Cooking Time: One hour and ten minutes

Yields: Four servings

Nutrition Facts: Calories: 687 | Protein: 27.9g | Carbs: 10.1g | Fat: 58.9g | Fiber: 6g

Ingredients

- Four legs of chicken
- Four tbsps. of olive oil
- Two tbsps. of Italian seasoning
- Pepper and salt
- Twenty ounces of each
    - Cherry tomatoes
    - Broccoli

For the garlic butter:

- Four ounces of butter
- Two cloves of garlic (smashed)
- Pepper and salt

Method

1. Toss the legs of the chicken with seasoning and oil.
2. Place the chicken legs in a baking sheet along with the tomatoes. Bake for forty-five minutes at 150 degrees Celsius.
3. As the chicken is cooking, cut the broccoli. Divide the florets and also slice the stem. Boil them in water for five minutes, along with some salt. Drain the broccoli water.
4. For making the garlic butter, combine all the ingredients in a small bowl.
5. Serve the cooked chicken legs with tomatoes, broccoli, and garlic butter by the side.

Note: Place the chicken legs in the oven with the skin side up.

Chapter 6: Staple Recipes

In this section, I have included some simple keto recipes made from everyday staples. Let's have a look at them.

Keto Waffles

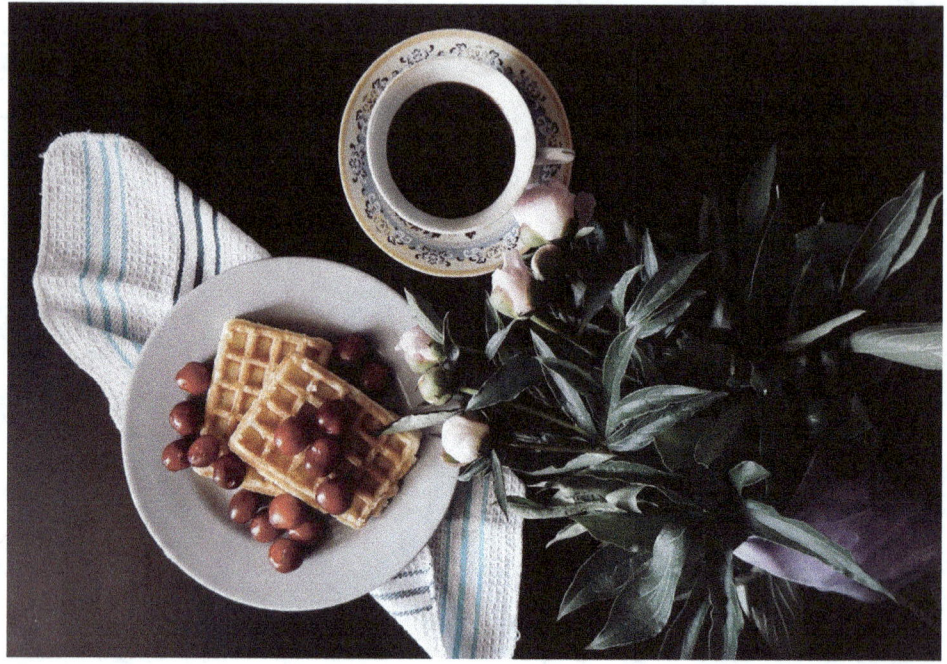

Total Prep & Cooking Time: Ten minutes

Yields: Two servings

Nutrition Facts: Calories: 160 | Protein: 21.3g | Carbs: 12.6g | Fat: 5.6g | Fiber: 10.3g

Ingredients

- Four tbsps. of coconut flour
- One tbsp. of each
    - Granulated sweetener

- - Apple sauce (unsweetened)
- One-fourth tsp. of each
  - Baking powder
  - Cinnamon
- Two-third cup of egg whites
- One-fourth cup of milk
- Half tsp. of vanilla extract
- One tsp. of coconut oil

Method:

1. Take a mixing bowl and mix the dry ingredients. Keep aside.

2. Add egg whites, vanilla extract, milk, and apple sauce in a bowl. Pour this mixture into the mixture of dry ingredients. Mix well.

3. Heat a waffle iron and grease with cooking spray or oil.

4. Add the waffle batter and cook for five minutes until fluffy and crisp.

Cookie Dough

Total Prep & Cooking Time: Ten minutes

Yields: Four servings

Nutrition Facts: Calories: 130 | Protein: 4.6g | Carbs: 4.3g | Fat: 12g | Fiber: 2.9g

Ingredients

- Half cup of almond flour
- Two tbsps. of each
    - Sticky sweetener
    - Granulated sweetener
    - Coconut flour
- One and a half tbsp. of coconut oil
- One tbsp. of chocolate chips

Method:

1. Combine coconut flour, almond flour, and granulated sugar in a bowl.
2. Add coconut oil and sticky sweetener. Mix well. Add the chocolate chips.
3. You can either enjoy the dough immediately or refrigerate it for thirty minutes.

Baked Tofu

Total Prep & Cooking Time: One hour and ten minutes

Yields: Two servings

Nutrition Facts: Calories: 131.3 | Protein: 11.3g | Carbs: 3.1g | Fat: 8.6g | Fiber: 1.7g

Ingredients

- One block of tofu (firm)
- One tbsp. of each
    - Soy sauce
    - Sesame oil
    - Tamari
- Half tsp. of each
    - Ginger
    - Garlic powder
    - Cayenne powder

Method:

1. Mix all the listed ingredients except for the tofu. Let the marinade sit for five minutes.

2. Chop the block of tofu into small pieces. Add the tofu cubes in the marinade. Refrigerate for half an hour.

3. Use parchment paper for lining a baking tray. Add the marinated tofu and bake for thirty minutes. Flip the tofu cubes halfway.

4. Serve immediately.

Cauliflower Fried Rice

Total Prep & Cooking Time: Twenty minutes

Yields: Four servings

Nutrition Facts: Calories: 135 | Protein: 7.9g | Carbs: 10.3g | Fat: 7.6g | Fiber: 8.6g

Ingredients

- Two tbsps. of sesame oil
- Two garlic cloves (finely chopped)
- One onion (finely chopped)
- Two scallions
- One-fourth cup of carrots (finely chopped)
- Eight cups of cauliflower rice
- Half cup of soy sauce
- One-fourth tsp. of cayenne pepper

Method:

1. Take a large wok and heat it over a medium flame. Addsome oil in it. Add garlic and onion. Cook for two minutes. Add scallions and carrots. Sauté for two minutes.

2. Add the cauliflower rice and combine well. Add cayenne and soy sauce. Fry for four minutes.

3. Serve the fried rice with scallions from the top.

PART II

Vegan Cookbook

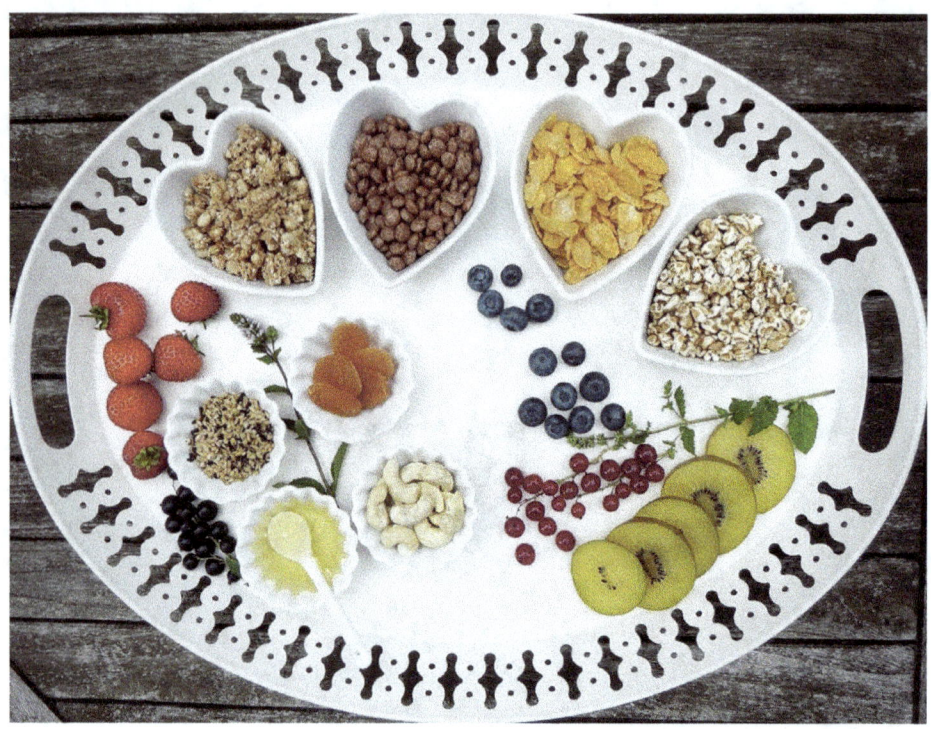

The vegan diet has gained immense popularity in the past few years. With an increasing number of participants, people have made up their mind to opt for the vegan options for health, environmental, or ethical reasons. When done in the perfect way, a vegan diet can help in showcasing a wide array of health benefits, for example, better control over blood sugar and a slimmer waistline. However, when a diet is based entirely on plant derivatives, it can result in a nutrient deficiency in various cases.

Veganism is being defined as a simple way of living that aims at excluding all major forms of animal cruelty and exploitation, whether for daily food, clothing, or some other purpose. For all these reasons, this diet does not include any form of animal products, such as eggs, dairy, and meat. It has been found that all those people who tend to practice veganism are thinner and also comes with a lower

BMI or body mass index when compared with non-vegans. This can easily explain the primary reason why the majority of the people are turning to this form of diet as the only way for losing extra weight.

Adopting a vegan diet can help keep the blood sugar level under proper check and type 2 diabetes. According to some studies, vegans tend to benefit from the lower levels of blood sugar, higher sensitivity to insulin, and about 77% lower risk of developing diabetes than the non-vegans. The majority of the advantages can be easily explained by the increased consumption of fiber, which can blunt the blood sugar response. Several observational studies reported that vegans could have a 74% lower risk of having increased blood pressure along with a 43% lower risk of suffering from any chronic heart disease.

There is a specific food group that you will need to omit for following a vegan diet. This group of foods includes:

- **Poultry and meat:** Lamb, beef, veal, pork, organ meat, chicken, wild meat, goose, turkey, duck, etc.

- **Dairy:** Yogurt, butter, milk, cheese, ice cream, cream, etc.

- **Seafood and fish:** Fish of all types, squid, anchovies, calamari, shrimp, lobster, mussels, crab, etc.

- **Eggs:** From ostrich, chicken, fish, quail, etc.

- **Products from bees:** Bee pollen, honey, royal jelly, etc.

- **Ingredients based on animals:** Casein, whey, egg white albumen, shellac, lactose, gelatin, L-cysteine, isinglass, omega-3 fatty acids derived from fish, vitamin D3 derived from animals, and carmine.

You can opt for alternatives such as legumes, seitan, tofu, seeds, nut butter, nuts, veggies, fruits, whole grains, etc. The cooking style will remain the same, and the only difference will be the ingredients you are going to use.

Chapter 1: Breakfast Recipes

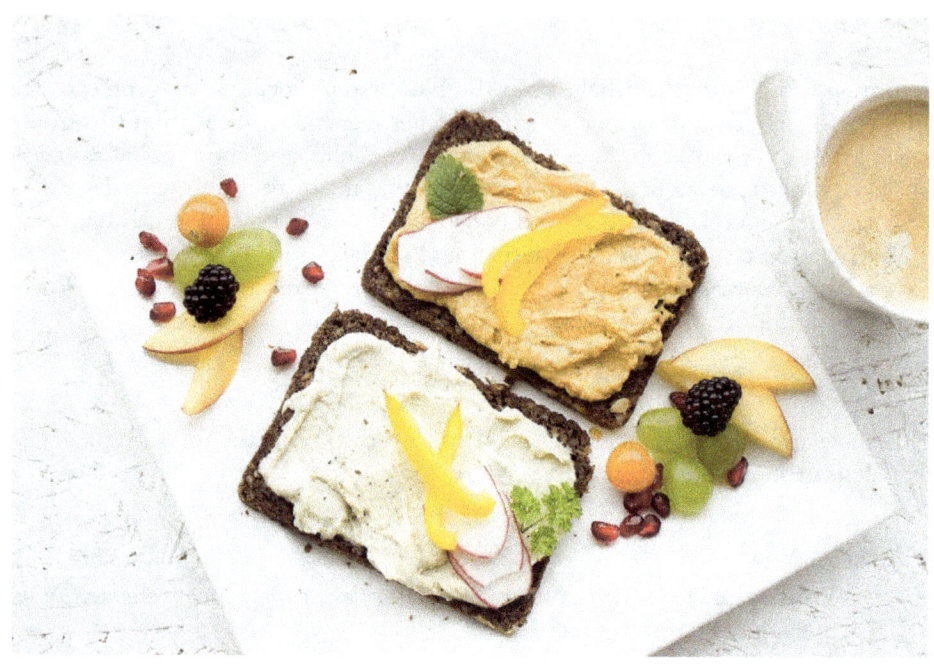

Breakfast is an essential meal of the day that needs to be fulfilled properly. Here are some vegan breakfast recipes for you.

Shamrock Sandwich
Total Prep & Cooking Time: Fifteen minutes

Yields: One serving

Nutrition Facts: Calories: 562 | Protein: 23g | Carbs: 43.2g | Fat: 31g | Fiber: 8.3g

Ingredients:

- One sausage patty (vegan)

- One cup of kale
- Two tsps. of olive oil (extra virgin)
- One tbsp. of pepitas
- Pepper and salt (according to taste)

For the sauce:

- One tbsp. of vegan mayonnaise
- One tsp. of jalapeno (chopped)
- One-fourth tsp. of paprika (smoky)

Other ingredients:

- One-fourth of an avocado (sliced)
- One toasted English muffin

Method:

1. Start by toasting the English muffin and keep it aside.

2. Take a sauté pan and drizzle some oil in it. Add the sausage patty and cook for two minutes on each side.

3. Add pepitas and kale to the hot pan. Add pepper and salt for adjusting the taste. When the kale gets soft, and the patty gets browned, remove the pan from heat.

4. Combine the spicy sauce.

5. Assemble the sandwich with sauce on the muffins and add the patty, avocado, pepitas, and kale.

Breakfast Burrito
Total Prep & Cooking Time: Thirty minutes

Yields: Two servings

Nutrition Facts: Calories: 618 | Protein: 20.3g | Carbs: 113g | Fat: 13.7g | Fiber: 21g

Ingredients:

- Three-fourth cup of rice (rinsed)
- Two cups of water
- One-fourth tsp. of salt
- One tbsp. of lime juice
- Half cup of cilantro (chopped)

For onions and hash browns:

- Half red onion
- Four red potatoes
- Two tbsp. of olive oil
- One-fourth tsp. of each
    - Black pepper (ground)
    - Salt

For black beans:

- One cup of black beans (cooked)
- One-fourth tsp. of each
    - Chili powder
    - Cumin powder
    - Garlic powder

For the avocado slaw:

- One avocado
- Two tbsps. of lime juice
- One cup of green cabbage (sliced thinly)
- One jalapeno (sliced)
- Half tsp. of each
    - Black pepper
    - Salt

For serving:

- Two flour tortillas
- Half avocado (ripe, sliced)
- One-fourth cup of salsa

Method:

1. Boil water, salt, and rice in a pan. Simmer the mixture for twenty minutes until the rice turns fluffy. Drain and keep aside.
2. Heat oil in a pan. Chop the potatoes into small pieces and slice the onions in rings. Add the potatoes along with the onions to the pan. Add pepper and salt for seasoning; toss the mixture for five minutes. Keep aside.
3. Prepare the beans in a saucepan over a medium flame.
4. For making the slaw, mix lime juice and avocado in a bowl. Mash the avocado and mix. Add jalapeno, cabbage, and toss for combining. Add pepper and salt for seasoning.
5. Add cilantro and lime juice to the rice and combine using a fork.
6. Warm the tortillas in a pan or microwave for twenty seconds.
7. Add the prepared fillings to the tortillas in order of your choice and top with salsa; add sliced avocado from the top. Roll the tortillas and slice in half.
8. Serve with extra black beans and potatoes by the side.

Gingerbread Waffles

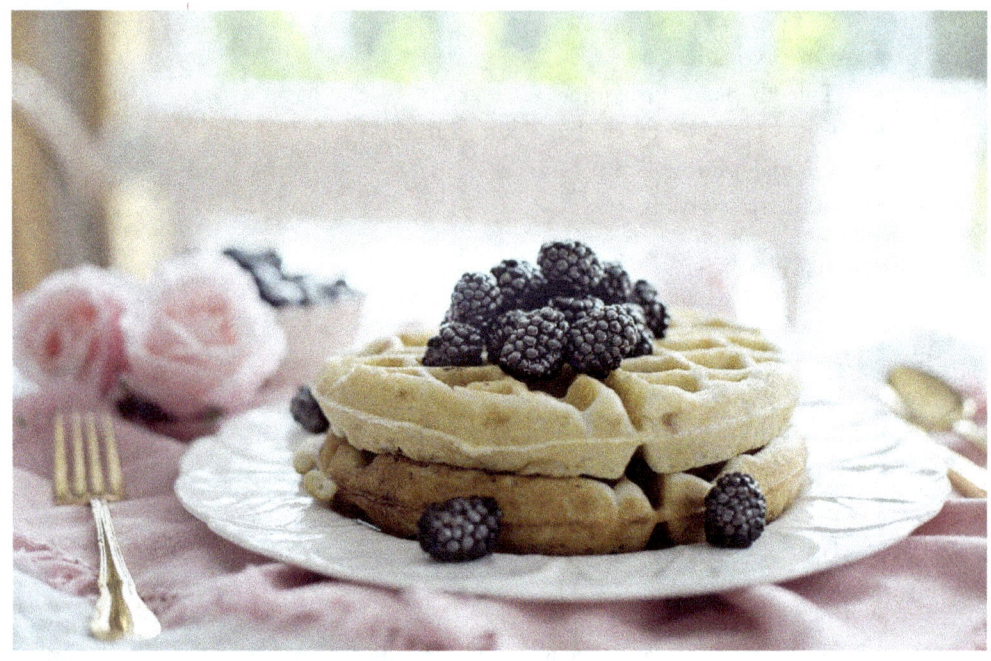

Total Prep & Cooking Time: Fifteen minutes

Yields: Six servings

Nutrition Facts: Calories: 170 | Protein: 4.2g | Carbs: 27.3g | Fat: 4.7g | Fiber: 3.9g

Ingredients:

- One cup of flour
- One tbsp. of flax seeds (ground)
- Two tsps. of baking powder
- One-fourth tsp. of each
    - Salt
    - Baking soda
- One tsp. of cinnamon (ground)

- One and a half tsps. of ginger (ground)
- Four tbsps. of brown sugar
- One cup of any non-dairy milk
- Two tbsps. of apple cider vinegar
- Two tbsps. of molasses
- One and a half tbsps. of olive oil

Method:

1. Preheat a waffle iron and grease it.
2. Put the dry ingredients in a mixing bowl and combine well.
3. Combine the wet ingredients in a medium mixing bowl or jug. Mix well until properly combined.
4. Add the mixture of wet ingredients into the dry mixture and mix well. The batter needs to be thick. In case the batter is excessively thick, you can add two tbsps. of non-dairy milk to the batter and mix.
5. Pour the batter in batches in the waffle iron and cook until steam stops to come out from the sides.
6. Open the waffle iron and take out the waffle carefully.
7. Serve warm.

Green Chickpeas And Toast

Total Prep & Cooking Time: Thirty minutes

Yields: Two servings

Nutrition Facts: Calories: 189 | Protein: 11.3g | Carbs: 27.1g | Fat: 3.2g | Fiber: 9.3g

Ingredients:

- Two tbsps. of olive oil
- Three shallots (diced)
- One-fourth tsp. of paprika (smoked)
- Two cloves of garlic (diced)
- Half tsp. of each
    - Sweet paprika
    - Salt
    - Cinnamon
    - Sugar
- Black pepper (according to taste)
- Two tomatoes (skinned)
- Two cups of chickpeas (cooked)
- Four crusty bread slices

Method:

1. Take a medium pan and heat oil in it.
2. Add the diced shallots to the oil and stir-fry. Add garlic to the pan. Cook for five minutes until shallots turn translucent.
3. Add spices to the pan and combine well with garlic and shallots. Stir for two minutes.
4. Add the tomatoes to the pan and squash them using a spoon or spatula. Add four tbsps. of water to the pan and simmer for twelve minutes.
5. Add cooked chickpeas and mix well. Add pepper, sugar, and salt.
6. Serve the cooked chickpeas on bread slices.

Asparagus And Tomato Quiche
Total Prep & Cooking Time: One hour and twenty minutes

Yields: Eight servings

Nutrition Facts: Calories: 219 | Protein: 4.1g | Carbs: 20.6g | Fat: 11.7g | Fiber: 3g

Ingredients:

- Two cups of flour
- Half tsp. of salt
- Half cup of non-dairy butter
- Two tbsps. of water (ice cold)

For filling:

- One tbsp. of coconut oil
- One cup of asparagus (chopped)
- One-fourth cup of onion (minced)
- Three tbsps. of each
    - Sun-dried tomatoes (chopped)
    - Nutritional yeast
    - Basil (chopped)
- One block of tofu (firm)
- One tbsp. of each
    - Flour
    - Non-dairy milk
- One tsp. of each
    - Minced onion (dehydrated)
    - Mustard
- Two tsps. of lemon juice
- Half tsp. of each
    - Salt
    - Turmeric
    - Liquid smoke

Method:

1. Spray a pie pan with oil and keep aside. Preheat your oven at 180 degrees Celsius.

2. Mix salt along with flour in a bowl. Add non-dairy butter along with cold water to the flour. Knead the dough on a working surface.

3. Press the dough on the pan. Bake the dough in the preheated oven for ten minutes.

4. Heat some oil in a pan and start adding asparagus, tomato, and onion— Cook for three minutes.

5. Combine onion, tofu, yeast, flour, non-dairy milk, lemon juice, liquid smoke, and salt in a blender.

6. Combine the mixture of asparagus with the tofu mixture.

7. Add the filling on the baked crust and smoothen the top.

8. Bake for half an hour.

9. Serve warm.

Breakfast Bowl

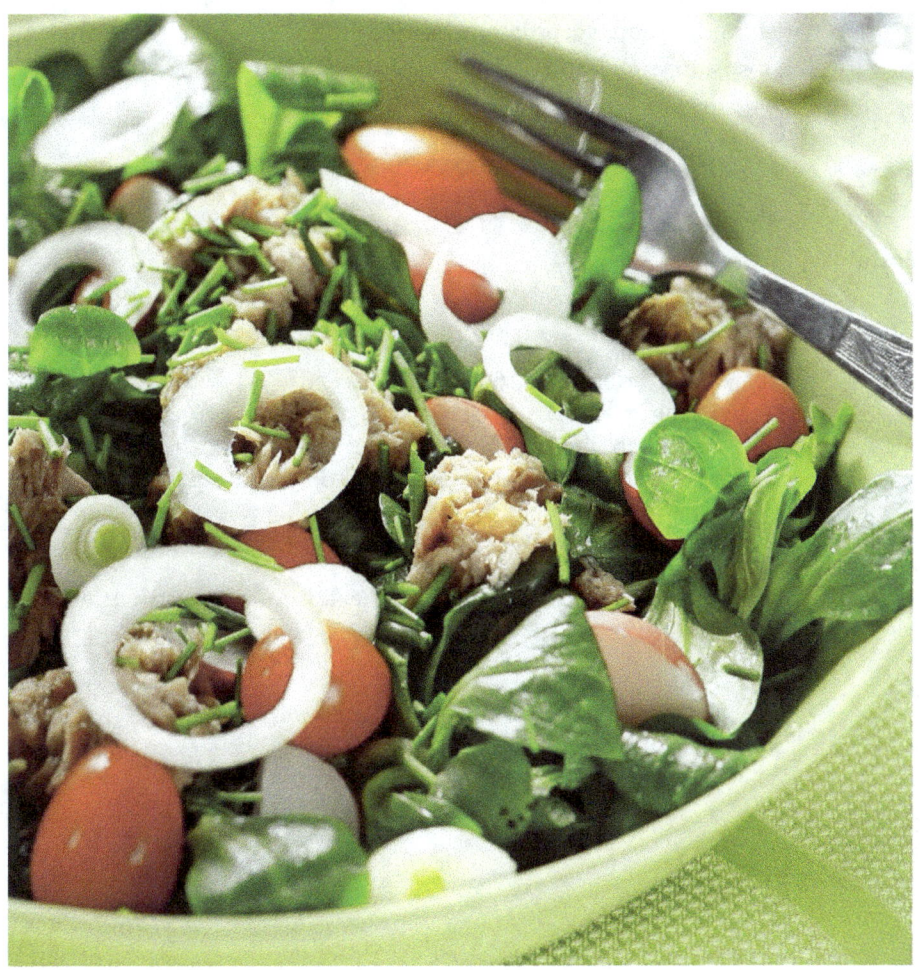

Total Prep & Cooking Time: One hour and twenty-five minutes

Yields: Two servings

Nutrition Facts: Calories: 350 | Protein: 7.2g | Carbs: 54g | Fat: 11.3g | Fiber: 9.3g

Ingredients:

- Two small sweet potatoes
- Cinnamon (ground, according to taste)
- Two tbsps. of each
    - Chopped nuts
    - Raisins
    - Almond butter

Method:

1. Preheat your oven at 180/160 degrees Celsius. Wash the potatoes and dry them using a kitchen towel. Use a fork for poking holes in the potatoes and wrap them using aluminum foil. Bake the potatoes for eighty minutes. Allow the potatoes to cool down before peeling.

2. Peel the baked potatoes and mash them with cinnamon.

3. Top with chopped nuts and raisins. Drizzle some almond butter from the top and serve.

Tofu Pancakes

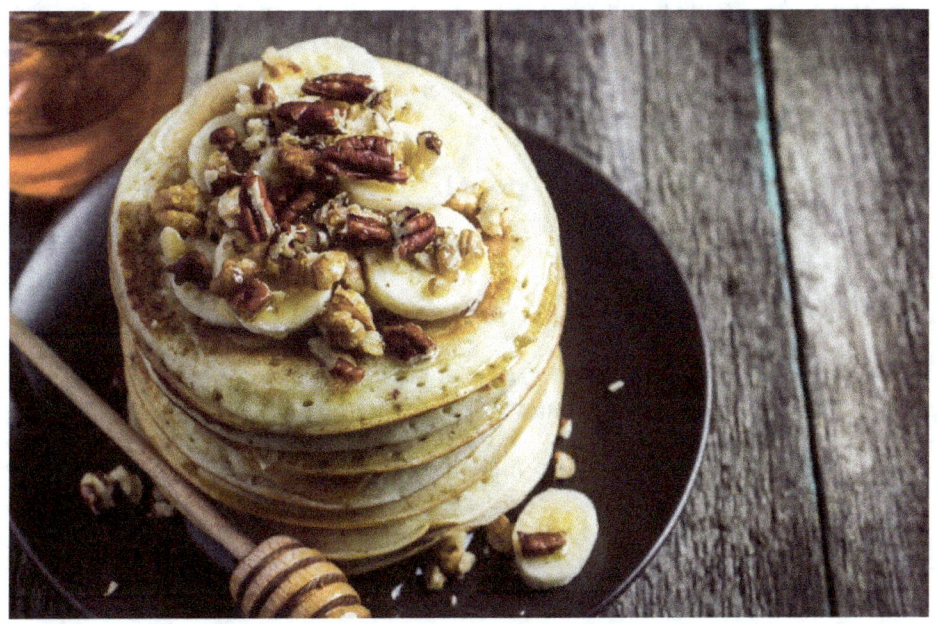

Total Prep & Cooking Time: Twenty minutes

Yields: Six servings

Nutrition Facts: Calories: 370 | Protein: 11.2g | Carbs: 46.3g | Fat: 13.2g | Fiber: 7.9g

Ingredients:

- Fifty grams of Brazil nuts
- Three bananas (sliced)
- Three-hundred grams of raspberries
- Maple syrup (for serving)

For batter:

- Four-hundred grams of firm tofu

- Two tsps. of each
    - Lemon juice
    - Vanilla extract
- Four-hundred ml of almond milk
- One tbsp. of vegetable oil
- Two cups of buckwheat flour
- Four tbsps. of sugar
- Two tsps. of mixed spice (ground)
- One tbsp. of baking powder

Method:

1. Preheat your oven at 160 degrees Celsius. Cook the nuts by scattering them in a tray for five minutes. Chop the nuts.

2. Add vanilla, tofu, almond milk, and lemon juice in a deep bowl; blend the mixture using a stick blender. Add oil to the mixture and blend again.

3. Take a large bowl and combine the dry ingredients; add one tsp. of salt and combine. Add the mixture of tofu and combine.

4. Heat a pan and add one tsp. oil in it. Make sure that the pan is not excessively hot.

5. Use a large spoon for dropping three spoons of batter in the pan. Swirl the pan for making the pancake even—Cook for two minutes on each side. Repeat the same for the remaining batter.

6. Serve with berries, bananas, nuts, and drizzle some maple syrup from the top.

Chapter 2: Side Dish Recipes

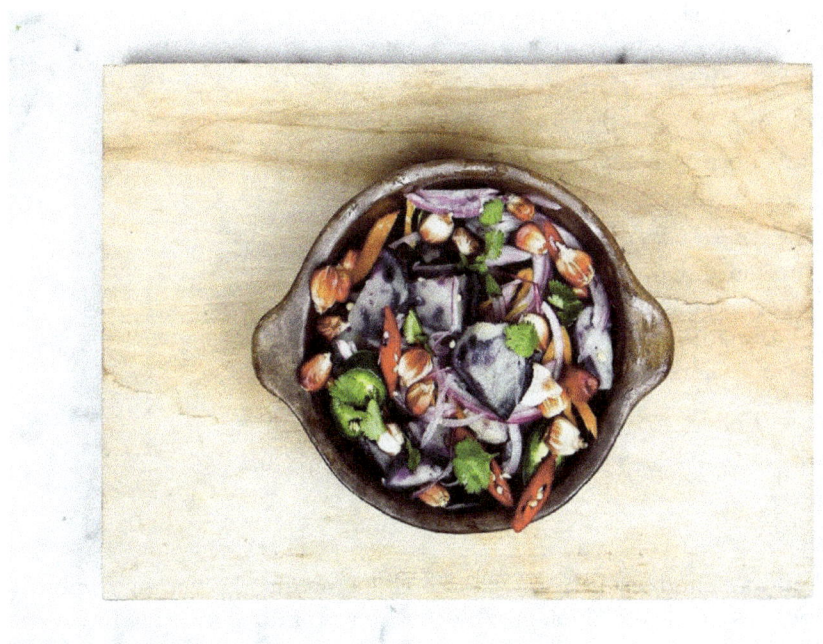

Side dish plays a profound role in any proper meal. I have included some tasty and easy vegan side dish recipes in this section.

Baked Beans
Total Prep & Cooking Time: Five hours and twenty minutes

Yields: Ten servings

Nutrition Facts: Calories: 249 | Protein: 11.2g | Carbs: 45.3g | Fat: 2.9g | Fiber: 13.7g

Ingredients:

- Sixteen ounces of navy beans (dry)

- Six cups of water
- Two tbsps. of olive oil
- Two cups of sweet onion (chopped)
- One garlic clove (minced)
- Four cans of tomato sauce
- One-fourth cup of brown sugar
- Half cup of molasses
- Three tbsps. of cider vinegar
- Three bay leaves
- One tsp. of mustard (dry)
- One-fourth tsp. of each
    - Black pepper (ground)
    - Nutmeg (ground)
    - Cinnamon (ground)

Method:

1. Add water and beans in a pot and boil the mixture. Lower the flame and cook for one hour. Cook until the beans are tender. Drain the beans and keep aside.

2. Preheat your oven to 160 degrees Celsius.

3. Take an iron skillet and heat oil in it. Add onions in the oil. Cook for two minutes. Add garlic to the pan.

4. Combine the onion mixture with the cooked beans. Add tomato sauce, molasses, vinegar, brown sugar, pepper, bay leaves, cinnamon, mustard, and nutmeg. Mix well.

5. Cover the dish and bake for three hours. Stir in between.

6. Remove the cover and bake for forty minutes.

Baked Potato Wedges
Total Prep & Cooking Time: Fifty-five minutes

Yields: Four servings

Nutrition Facts: Calories: 234 | Protein: 5.1g | Carbs: 42.6g | Fat: 4.3g | Fiber: 8.9g

Ingredients:

- One tbsp. of olive oil
- Eight sweet potatoes (sliced into quarters)
- Half tsp. of paprika

Method:

1. Preheat your oven at 160/180 degrees Celsius.
2. Grease a baking sheet with cooking spray.
3. Combine potatoes and paprika in a bowl. Add the potatoes to the baking sheet.
4. Bake for forty minutes.
5. Serve warm.

Black Beans And Quinoa

Total Prep & Cooking Time: Fifty minutes

Yields: Ten servings

Nutrition Facts: Calories: 143 | Protein: 8.7g | Carbs: 25.6g | Fat: 1.2g | Fiber: 8.7g

Ingredients:

- One tsp. of vegetable oil
- One large onion (chopped)
- Three garlic cloves (chopped)
- Three-fourth cup of quinoa
- Two cups of vegetable stock
- One tsp. of cumin (ground)
- One-fourth tsp. of cayenne powder
- One cup of corn kernels (frozen)
- Two cans of black beans (rinsed)
- Half cup of cilantro (chopped)
- Pepper and salt (according to taste)

Method:

1. Take a medium pan and heat oil in it. Add garlic and onion to the pan. Cook for ten minutes until browned.

2. Add quinoa to the pan and mix well. Cover the mixture with vegetable stock. Season with salt, pepper, and cayenne. Boil the mixture. Cover the pan and simmer for twenty minutes until quinoa gets tender.

3. Add the corn kernels to the pan and simmer for five minutes.

4. Add cilantro and black beans to the mixture.

5. Serve hot.

Roasted Lemon Garlic Broccoli

Total Prep & Cooking Time: Twenty-five minutes

Yields: Six servings

Nutrition Facts: Calories: 48.3 | Protein: 3g | Carbs: 6.9g | Fat: 1.8g | Fiber: 3g

Ingredients:

- Two heads of broccoli (separate the florets)
- Two tsps. of olive oil (extra virgin)
- One tsp. of salt
- Half tsp. of black pepper (ground)
- One garlic clove (minced)
- One-fourth tsp. of lemon juice

Method:

1. Preheat your oven at 180/200 degrees Celsius.
2. Toss the florets of broccoli with olive oil in a bowl. Add pepper, garlic, and salt. Spread the coated broccoli florets on a baking sheet.
3. Bake for twenty minutes.
4. Add lemon juice from the top and serve warm.

Spicy Tofu

Total Prep & Cooking Time: Twenty minutes

Yields: Four servings

Nutrition Facts: Calories: 305.2 | Protein: 20.1g | Carbs: 15.4g | Fat: 19.3g | Fiber: 5.2g

Ingredients:

- Three tbsps. of peanut oil
- One red onion (sliced)
- One pound of tofu (firm, cubed)
- One bell pepper (sliced)
- One chili pepper (chopped)
- Three garlic cloves (crushed)
- One-third cup of hot water
- Two tbsps. of each
    - Soy sauce
    - White vinegar
- One tsp. of cornstarch
- One tbsp. of each
    - Red pepper flakes (crushed)
    - Brown sugar

Method:

1. Take a wok and heat oil in it. Add the tofu to the oil and keep cooking until browned. Add bell pepper, onion, garlic, and chili pepper. Mix well and cook for five minutes.

2. Whisk vinegar, soy sauce, red pepper flakes, brown sugar, and cornstarch in a bowl.

3. Add the mixture of vinegar to the wok and toss well for coating. Simmer the mixture for five minutes.

4. Serve hot.

Spanish Rice
Total Prep & Cooking Time: Forty minutes

Yields: Four servings

Nutrition Facts: Calories: 267.2 | Protein: 4.7g | Carbs: 42.7g | Fat: 5.6g | Fiber: 3g

Ingredients:

- Two tbsps. of vegetable oil
- One cup of white rice (uncooked)
- One onion (chopped)
- Half bell pepper (chopped)
- Two cups of water
- One can of green chilies and diced tomatoes
- Two tsps. of chili powder
- One tsp. of salt

Method:

1. Take a deep skillet and heat oil in it. Add onion, rice, and bell pepper to the skillet. Sauté until onions are soft and rice gets browned.

2. Add tomatoes and water to the skillet. Add salt and chili powder.

3. Simmer the mixture for thirty minutes and cover the skillet.

4. Serve hot.

Pepper And Lemon Pasta

Total Prep & Cooking Time: Twenty minutes

Yields: Eight servings

Nutrition Facts: Calories: 232.8 | Protein: 8.5g | Carbs: 41g | Fat: 4.6g | Fiber: 3.6g

Ingredients:

- One pound of spaghetti
- Two tbsps. of olive oil
- One tbsp. of basil (dried)
Three tbsps. of lemon juice
- Black pepper (ground, according to taste)

Method:

1. Take a large pot and boil water in it with light salt. Add the pasta to the pot and cook for ten minutes. Drain the pasta.

2. Combine lemon juice, black pepper, lemon juice, and basil in a bowl.

3. Add the lemon mixture to the cooked pasta and toss it properly.

4. Serve cold or hot

Chapter 3: High Protein Recipes

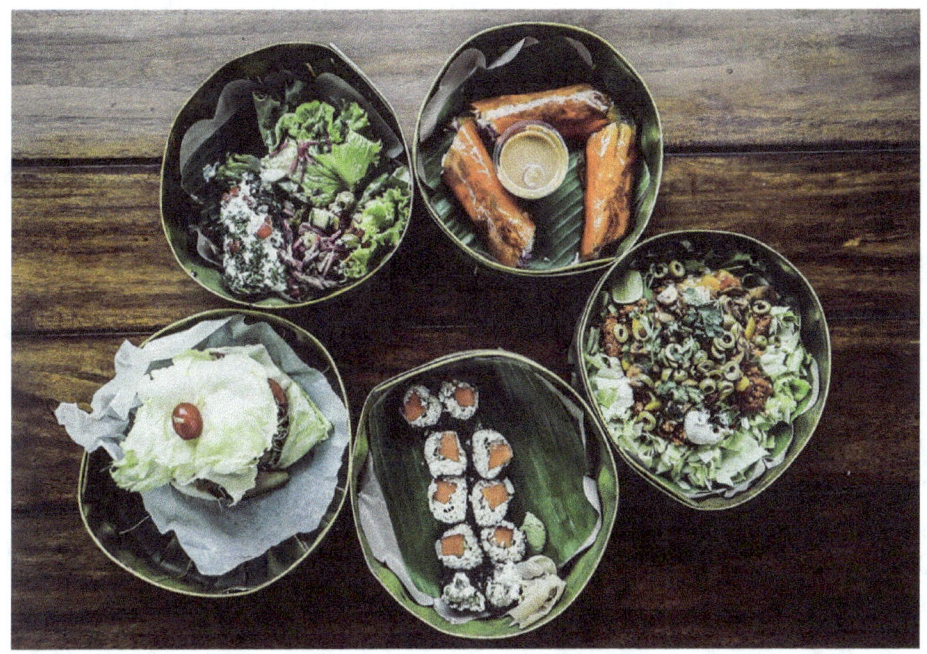

The vegan diet is rich in proteins, as it is mainly composed of plant compounds. Here are some easy to make vegan high protein recipes for you.

Kale Salad With Spicy Tempeh Bits And Chickpeas

Total Prep & Cooking Time: Forty-five minutes

Yields: Four servings

Nutrition Facts: Calories: 473 | Protein: 25g | Carbs: 41g | Fat: 27.1g | Fiber: 17.3g

Ingredients:

- Eight ounces of tempeh
- One-fourth cup of vegetable oil
- One-fourth tsp. of salt
- Two tsps. of each
    - Garlic powder

- - Onion powder
    - Sweet paprika
- One tsp. of each
    - Lemon pepper
    - Chili powder
- One-eighth tsp. of cayenne powder

For salad:

- 400 grams of kale (chopped)
- One cup of carrots (shredded)
- One can of chickpeas
- Two tbsps. of sesame seeds

For dressing:

- Half cup of rice vinegar
- One-fourth cup of soy sauce
- Two tbsps. of sesame oil
- One tbsp. of ginger (grated)

Method:

1. Boil water with salt in a large pot. Blanch the kale for thirty seconds. Wash blanched kale under running water. Squeeze out excess water from kale and keep aside.

2. Preheat your oven to 180 degrees Celsius.

3. Mix all the spices for tempeh in a mixing bowl.

4. Cut tempeh into very thin slices.

5. Dip each tempeh slice in oil and arrange them on a baking sheet. Line the tray using parchment paper. Sprinkle the mix of spices from the top. Coat well.

6. Bake tempeh for twenty minutes until crispy and brown in color.

7. Take a large bowl and combine the listed ingredients for the salad.

8. Combine the ingredients of dressing in a jar and shake well.

9. Pour the dressing over the prepared salad. Toss well. Make sure the salad gets coated properly with the dressing.

10. Crumble the slices of tempeh over the salad.

Protein Bars
Total Prep & Cooking Time: One hour and twenty minutes

Yields: Ten servings

Nutrition Facts: Calories: 292 | Protein: 13g | Carbs: 37.9g | Fat: 9.6g | Fiber: 2.3g

Ingredients:

For crust:

- Two cups of oat flour
- Six apricots (dried)
- One-fourth cup of each
    - Brown rice syrup
    - Cocoa powder

For layer:

- One cup of oat flour
- Half cup of each
    - Vegan protein powder (chocolate)
    - Rolled oats
- One-fourth tsp. of salt
- Two tbsps. of each
    - Hemp seeds (hulled)
    - Chia seeds
- Half cup of almond butter
- One-fourth cup of any vegan sweetener
- One cup of coconut milk
- One tbsp. flax seeds (ground)

Method:

1. Combine all the ingredients for the crust in a blender. Keep the dough aside.

2. Take a large bowl and mix the dry ingredients for the next layer. You can use a fork for proper mixing.

3. Mix water and flax in a bowl and keep aside until it turns into a gel.

4. Add almond butter, sweetener, coconut milk, and flax gel to the mixture of dry ingredients. Use a fork for mixing properly.

5. Pour the mixture in a food processor and blend well for making it smooth.

6. Use parchment paper for lining a baking sheet. Add the crust to the sheet and press the crust out. Add the next layer on the crust and evenly spread it out.

7. Put the baking sheet in the freezer for one hour.

8. Serve by cutting bars of your desired size and shape.

Tofu And Spinach Scramble

Total Prep & Cooking Time: Thirty minutes

Yields: Two servings

Nutrition Facts: Calories: 319 | Protein: 22.1g | Carbs: 11.4g | Fat: 22g | Fiber: 6.5g

Ingredients:

- Fourteen ounces of tofu (firm, cut into cubes of half-inch)
- Half tsp. of turmeric (ground)
- Black pepper and kosher salt (to taste)
- One-eighth tsp. of cayenne powder (ground)
- Two tbsps. of olive oil (extra virgin)
- Three scallions (sliced)
- Five ounces of spinach (chopped)
- Two tsps. of lemon juice
- One cup of grape tomatoes (halved)
- Half cup of basil (chopped)

Method:

1. Mix turmeric, tofu, one-fourth tsp. of salt, cayenne, and half tsp. of black pepper in a bowl. Toss the ingredients for mixing properly.

2. Take a large skillet and heat oil in it; add the scallions and stir for about one minute. Add tofu mixture and cook for five minutes until the tofu gets browned.

3. Add lemon juice, spinach, and half tsp. of salt to the tofu. Cook for one minute until the spinach wilts. Add tomatoes and stir for one minute.

4. Remove the skillet from heat and add basil.

5. Serve hot.

Vegan Tacos

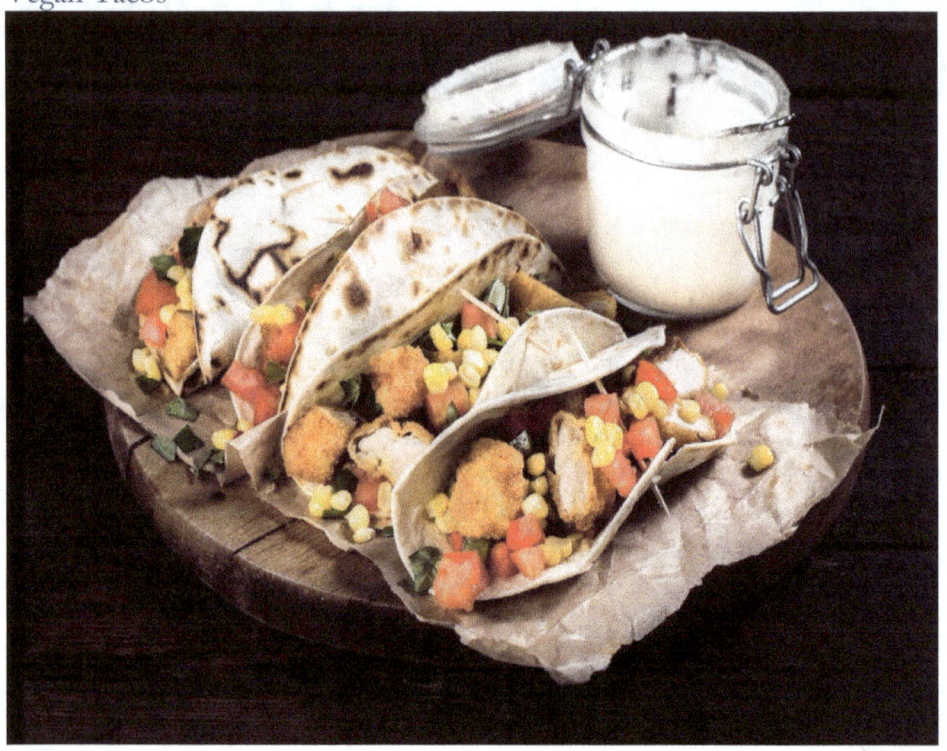

Total Prep & Cooking Time: Twenty minutes

Yields: Six servings

Nutrition Facts: Calories: 402 | Protein: 29g | Carbs: 71.2g | Fat: 5.4g | Fiber: 20.3g

Ingredients:

- One tsp. of vegetable oil
- Half onion (diced)
- Two tsps. of jalapeno (chopped)
- Twelve ounces of soy chorizo (remove the casing)
- Sixteen ounces of refried black beans

- Twelve tortillas (corn)
- Cilantro (chopped)

Method:

1. Take a skillet and heat oil in it. Add onion and jalapeno to the skillet—Cook for ten minutes. Add chorizo and cook for five minutes.
2. Take a small pan and cook the beans on low heat.
3. Arrange two tortillas for making six tacos in total.
4. Spread the beans on the tortillas; top the beans with the mixture of chorizo. Serve with cilantro from the top.

Grilled Tofu Steaks And Spinach Salad

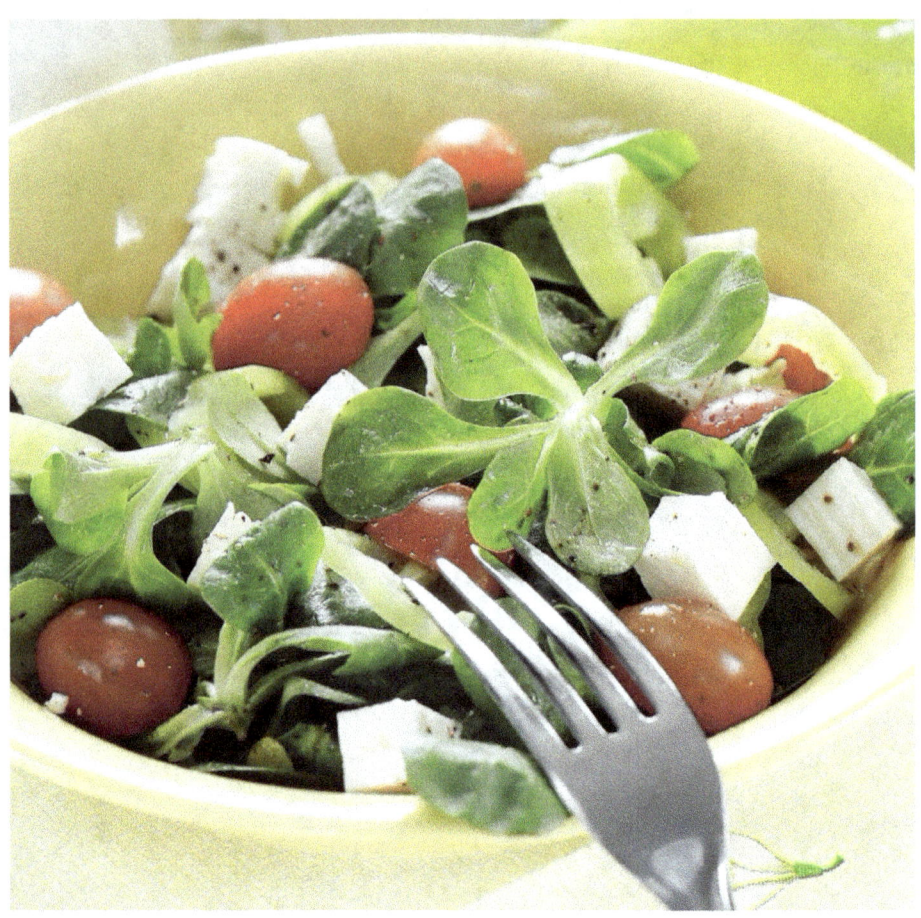

Total Prep & Cooking Time: One hour

Yields: Two servings

Nutrition Facts: Calories: 154 | Protein: 22g | Carbs: 8g | Fat: 11.3g | Fiber: 9.3g

Ingredients:

For tofu steak:

- Half block of tofu (firm)
- One tbsp. of soy sauce
- One tsp. of each
    - Miso paste
    - Tomato paste
    - Olive oil
- Half tsp. of maple syrup
- One-fourth cup of breadcrumbs

For spinach salad:

- Two cups of baby spinach
- One tbsp. of each
    - Olive oil (extra virgin)
    - Pine nuts
    - Lemon juice
- Pinch of salt
- Pinch of black pepper (ground)

Method:

1. Cut the tofu block in half and squeeze out any excess water. Make sure you do not break the block of tofu. Use paper towels for drying the tofu.

2. Cut the tofu in size and shape of your choice.

3. Take a small mixing bowl and combine tomato paste, soy sauce, olive oil, sesame, miso paste, and maple syrup. Mix until the sauce is smooth.

4. Spread breadcrumbs in a shallow dish.

5. Dip the pieces of tofu in the prepared sauce and then coat them in breadcrumbs. Repeat for the remaining tofu.

6. Grease a grill pan with some olive oil. Add the tofu steaks and cook for fifteen minutes on each side. Cook until both sides are browned.

7. For the salad, mix the listed ingredients in a medium-sized mixing bowl. Toss the ingredients properly.

8. Serve the tofu steaks with spinach salad by the side.

Corn, Quinoa, And Edamame Salad
Total Prep & Cooking Time: Two hours and ten minutes

Yields: Four servings

Nutrition Facts: Calories: 130 | Protein: 18g | Carbs: 13g | Fat: 5.8g | Fiber: 3.1g

Ingredients:

- One cup of corn kernels (frozen)
- Two cups of shelled edamame
- Half cup of cooked quinoa
- One green onion (sliced)
- Half sweet bell pepper (diced)
- Two tbsps. of cilantro (chopped)
- One and a half tbsps. of olive oil
- One tbsp. of each
    - Lime juice
    - Lemon juice
- One-fourth tsp. of each
    - Salt
    - Thyme (dried)
    - Chili powder
    - Black pepper (ground)

Method:

1. Boil corn and edamame in water with a little bit of salt. Drain and keep aside.

2. Take a bowl and mix corn, edamame, quinoa, bell pepper, green onion, and cilantro.

3. Whisk together lemon juice, olive oil, lime juice, chili powder, salt, thyme, and black pepper in a small bowl.

4. Pour the dressing all over the salad. Mix well.

5. Chill in the refrigerator for two hours.

Lentil Soup

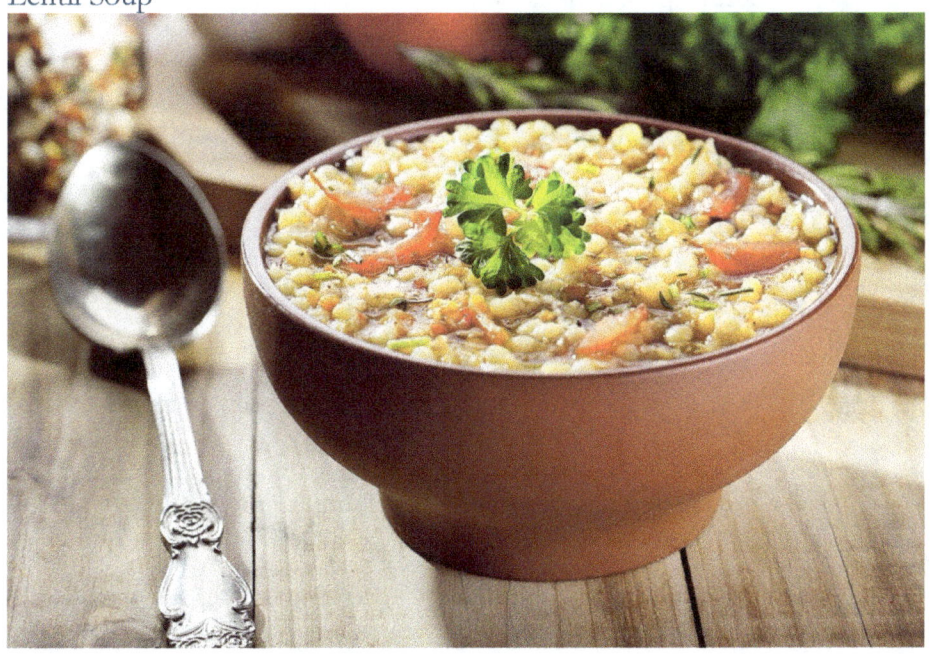

Total Prep & Cooking Time: Fifty-five minutes

Yields: Six servings

Nutrition Facts: Calories: 230 | Protein: 9.2g | Carbs: 31.2g | Fat: 8.6g | Fiber: 11.3g

Ingredients:

- Two tbsps. of olive oil (extra virgin)
- One onion (diced)
- Two carrots (diced)
- Two stalks of celery (diced)
- One bell pepper (diced)
- Three garlic cloves (minced)
- One tbsp. of cumin

- One-fourth tsp. of paprika
- One tsp. of oregano
- Two cups of tomatoes (diced)
- Two cans of green lentils (rinsed)
- Eight cups of vegetable stock
- Half tsp. of salt
- Cilantro (for garnishing)
- One ripe avocado (diced)

Method:

1. Heat some oil in a pot. Start adding bell pepper, onion, carrots, and celery to the pot. Sauté the veggies for five minutes until tender; add paprika, cumin, garlic, and oregano. Mix well.

2. Add chilies, tomatoes, stock, salt, and lentils; simmer the mixture for forty minutes. Add pepper and salt according to taste.

3. Serve with avocado and cilantro from the top.

Chapter 4: Dessert Recipes

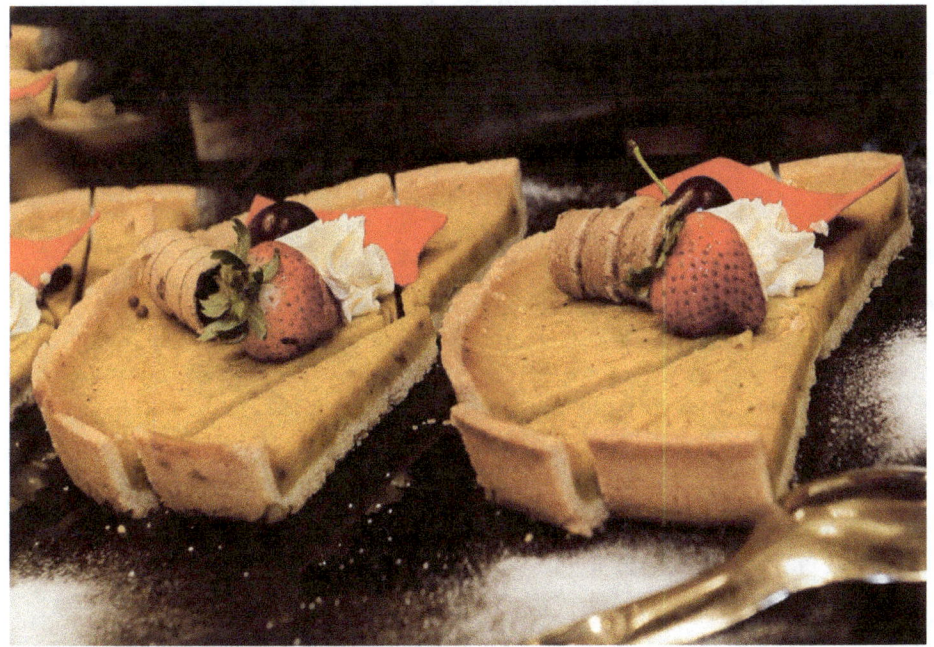

Everyone loves to have some dessert after having their meals. Desserts can be vegan too. So in this section, I have included some tasty dessert recipes that you can make easily.

Chocolate Pudding
Total Prep & Cooking Time: Forty-five minutes

Yields: Two servings

Nutrition Facts: Calories: 265.1 | Protein: 8.3g | Carbs: 52.2g | Fat: 4.6g | Fiber: 4.9g

Ingredients:

- Three tbsps. of cornstarch
- Two tbsps. of water

- Two cups of soy milk
- One-fourth tsp. of vanilla extract
- One-fourth cup of white sugar
- One cup of cocoa powder

Method:

1. Take a small bowl and mix water and cornstarch for forming a fine paste.
2. Take a saucepan and heat it over medium flame. Add soy milk, sugar, vanilla, a mixture of cornstarch, and cocoa. Stir the mixture until it starts boiling. Keep cooking until the mixture gets thick.
3. Allow the pudding to cool for five minutes.
4. Chill in the fridge for twenty minutes.

Orange Cake

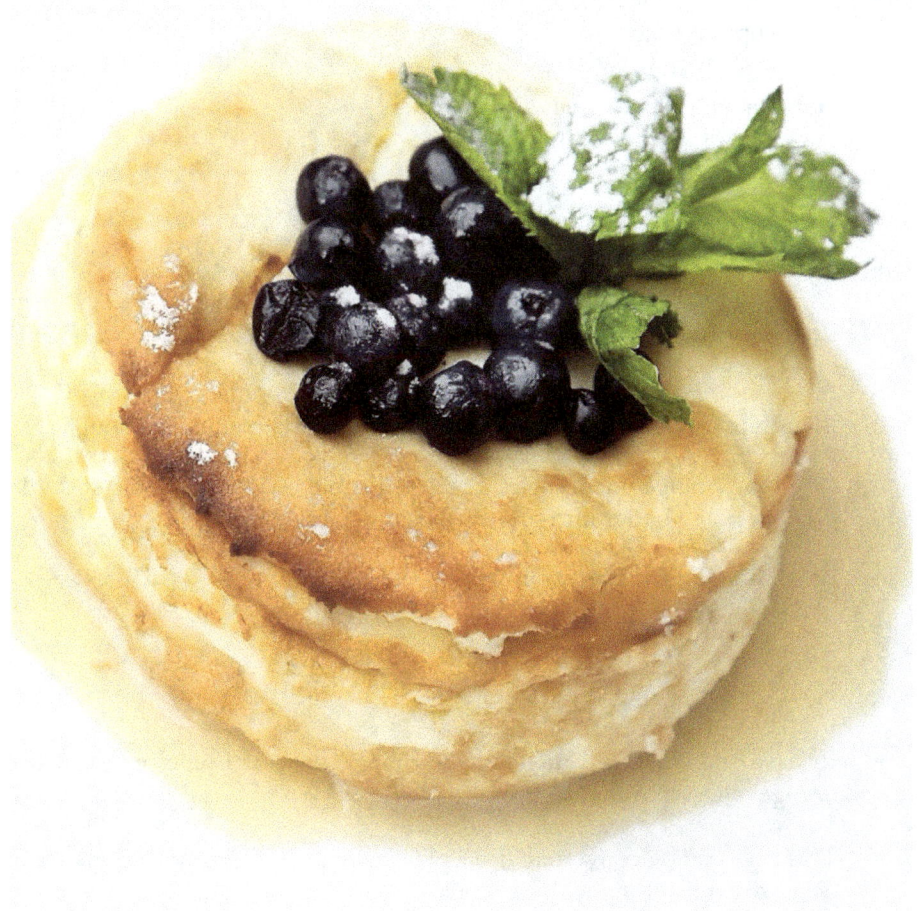

Total Prep & Cooking Time: Forty-five minutes

Yields: Sixteen servings

Nutrition Facts: Calories: 147.3 | Protein: 1.9g | Carbs: 21.6g | Fat: 6.3g | Fiber: 0.8g

Ingredients:

- One large-sized onion (peeled)
- Two cups of flour
- One cup of white sugar
- Half cup of vegetable oil
- One and a half tsps. of baking soda
- Half tsp. of salt

Method:

1. Preheat your oven to 190 degrees Celsius. Grease a baking pan with some oil.

2. Blend the orange in a food processor until it gets completely liquefied.

3. Combine orange juice, sugar, flour, vegetable oil, baking soda, and salt. Pour the cake batter into prepared baking pan.

4. Bake the cake for thirty minutes.

Notes:

- In case you do not want to make orange juice at home, you can use orange juice from the store.

- This cake can be converted into a plain cake by omitting orange juice and using soy milk along with rice milk.

Pumpkin Tofu Pie

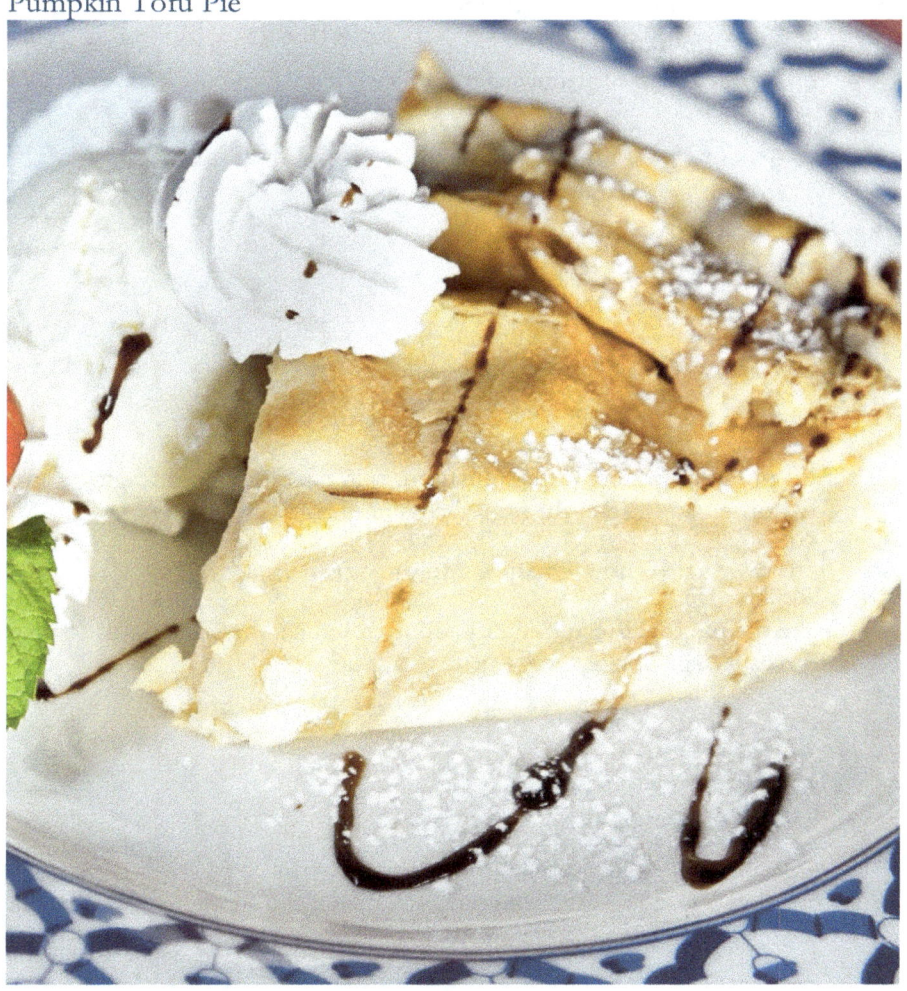

Total Prep & Cooking Time: Two hours

Yields: Eight servings

Nutrition Facts: Calories: 229.3 | Protein: 4.7g | Carbs: 33.6g | Fat: 8.6g | Fiber: 3.7g

Ingredients

- Ten ounces of silken tofu (drained)
- One can of pumpkin puree
- Three-fourth cup of white sugar
- Half tsp. of salt
- One tsp. of cinnamon (ground)
- One-fourth tsp. of ginger (ground)
- One-eighth tsp. of cloves (ground)
- One pie crust (unbaked)

Method:

1. Preheat the oven at 220/230 degrees Celsius.

2. Add pumpkin puree, tofu, cinnamon, salt, sugar, clove, and ginger in a food processor. Blend the ingredients until smooth.

3. Pour over the blended mixture into the crust.

4. Bake the pie for fifteen minutes and then reduce the temperature to 175 degrees Celsius. Bake again for forty minutes.

5. Let the pie cool down.

6. Serve at room temperature.

Note: If you are allergic to certain ingredients, check the ingredients of the pie crust.

Vegan Brownie

Total Prep & Cooking Time: Fifty minutes

Yields: Sixteen servings

Nutrition Facts: Calories: 254.3 | Protein: 2.6g | Carbs: 38.3g | Fat: 13.6g | Fiber: 2.8g

Ingredients:

- Two cups of flour
- Two cups of white sugar
- Three-fourth cup of cocoa powder (unsweetened)
- One tsp. of baking powder
- Half tsp. of salt
- One cup of each
    - Vegetable oil
    - Water
- One and a half tsps. of vanilla extract

Method:

1. Preheat your oven at 160/175 degrees Celsius.
2. Take a large bowl and combine sugar, flour, cocoa powder, salt, and baking powder. Add vegetable oil, vanilla extract, and water to the mixture. Mix well for making a smooth batter.
3. Spread the brownie mix in a baking pan.
4. Bake the brownie for thirty minutes.
5. Allow the brownie to cool for ten minutes.
6. Cut in squares and serve.

Vegan Cupcake

Total Prep & Cooking Time: Twenty-five minutes

Yields: Eighteen servings

Nutrition Facts: Calories: 150.2 | Protein: 1.9g | Carbs: 21.6g | Fat: 6.3g | Fiber: 0.9g

Ingredients:

- One tbsp. of cider vinegar
- Two cups of almond milk
- Two and a half cups of flour
- One cup of white sugar
- Two tsps. of baking powder
- Half tsp. of each
    - Salt
    - Baking soda
    - Coconut oil (warmed)
- One and a half tsps. of vanilla extract

Method:

1. Preheat the oven at 160/175 degrees Celsius. Grease eighteen muffin cups using some oil.

2. Mix cider vinegar and almond milk in a bowl. Allow it to stand for five minutes until the mixture gets curdled.

3. Take a bowl and combine sugar, salt, baking powder, flour, and baking soda.

4. Take another bowl and combine coconut oil, vanilla, and almond milk mixture. Add this mixture to the mixture of dry ingredients.

5. Divide the batter into muffin cups—Bake for twenty minutes.

6. Allow the cupcakes to sit for ten minutes.

7. Serve with the desired frosting from the top.

Vanilla Cake

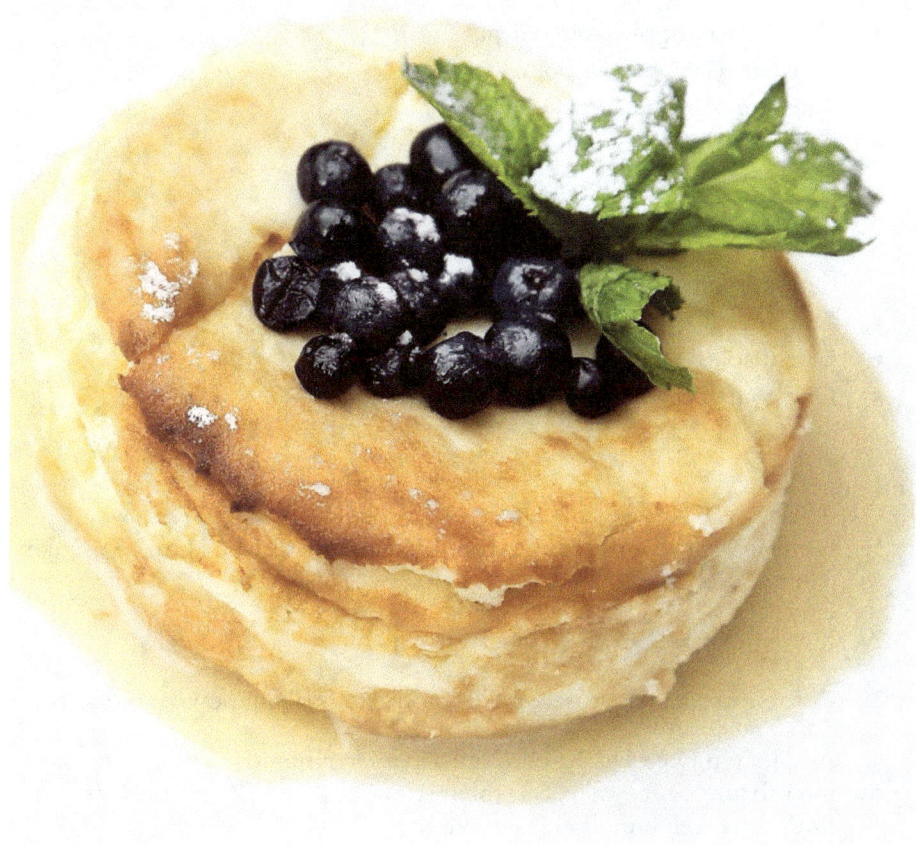

Total Prep & Cooking Time: Fifty minutes

Yields: Eight servings

Nutrition Facts: Calories: 277.9 | Protein: 3.5g | Carbs: 44.2g | Fat: 9.2g | Fiber: 0.9g

Ingredients:

- One cup of soy milk
- One tbsp. of apple cider vinegar
- One and a half cup of flour
- One cup of white sugar
- One tsp. of each
    - Baking powder
    - Baking soda
- Half tsp. of salt
- One-third cup of canola oil
- One-fourth tsp. of almond extract
- One tbsp. of vanilla extract
- One-fourth cup of water

Method:

1. Preheat your oven at about 160/175 degrees Celsius. Grease a baking pan with some oil.

2. Mix vinegar and soy milk in a large cup.

3. Combine sugar, flour, salt, baking soda, and baking powder in a bowl.

4. Add lemon juice, canola oil, vanilla extract, almond extract, and water to the mixture of soy milk. Stir the mixture of soy milk into the mixture of flour. Mix well until there is no lump.

5. Pour the cake batter in the baking dish.

6. Bake in the preheated oven for thirty-five minutes.

Miracle Fudge
Total Prep & Cooking Time: One hour and ten minutes

Yields: Twenty-four servings

Nutrition Facts: Calories: 77.3 | Protein: 0.9g | Carbs: 4.9g | Fat: 6.2g | Fiber: 1.2g

Ingredients:

- Half cup of cocoa (unsweetened)
- One cup of maple syrup
- One tsp. of vanilla extract
- One pinch of salt
- One-third cup of each
    - Chopped walnuts
    - Coconut oil (melted)
- One tsp. of cocoa powder (unsweetened, for dusting)

Method

1. Add half cup of cocoa powder in a bowl along with maple syrup; give it a stir. Add vanilla extract and salt. Add melted coconut oil and combine well.

2. Add walnuts in a pan and toast them for one minute.

3. Add the toasted walnuts to the fudge. Mix well.

4. Pour the mixture of fudge into a silicone mold. Smoothen the top.

5. Wrap the silicone mold using plastic wrap and put it in the freezer for thirty minutes. Take out the fudge pieces from the mold and dust with cocoa powder from the top.

6. Serve cold.

Chapter 5: Sauces & Dips Recipes

Sauces and dips are important components of any meal that can make the food tastier. Here are some vegan sauces and dips recipes for you.

Tomato Jam
Total Prep & Cooking Time: Forty-five minutes

Yields: One full cup

Nutrition Facts: Calories: 34 | Protein: 0.2g | Carbs: 8.6g | Fat: 0.1g | Fiber: 0.2g

Ingredients:

- Two pounds of plum tomatoes
- One-fourth cup of coconut sugar
- Half tsp. of salt
- One-fourth tsp. of paprika
- One tsp. of vinegar (white wine)
- Black pepper (to taste)

Method:

1. Take a large pot and boil water in it; add the tomatoes to the water and boil for one minute. Remove the tomatoes and put them in an ice-water bath.

2. Peel the blanched tomatoes and chop them.

3. Add chopped tomatoes in a pot over a medium flame. Add sugar and stir the mixture—Cook for ten minutes.

4. Add pepper, salt, and paprika. Simmer for ten minutes until the jam thickens.

5. Remove from heat and add white wine vinegar. Serve with crackers, burgers, toasts, etc.

Walnut Kale Pesto
Total Prep & Cooking Time: Thirty minutes

Yields: One small bowl

Nutrition Facts: Calories: 240 | Protein: 3.6g | Carbs: 2.6g | Fat: 22.3g | Fiber: 0.8g

Ingredients:

- Half bunch of kale (chopped)
- Half cup of walnuts (chopped)
- Two garlic cloves (minced)
- One-fourth cup of yeast
- One cup of olive oil
- Three tbsps. of lemon juice
- Pepper and salt (for seasoning)

Method:

1. Take a pot and boil water in it. Add kale to the pot with one tsp. of salt— Cook for five minutes.

2. Add kale, garlic, walnuts, olive oil, yeast, along with lemon juice in a food processor. Add pepper and salt according to your taste. Blend well.

Ranch Dressing

Total Prep & Cooking Time: Thirty minutes

Yields: One small bowl

Nutrition Facts: Calories: 92 | Protein: 0.1g | Carbs: 1g | Fat: 9.1g | Fiber: 0.4g

Ingredients:

- One cup of vegan mayo
- Half tsp. of each
    - Onion powder
    - Garlic powder
- One-fourth tsp. of black pepper (ground)
- Two tsps. of parsley (chopped)
- One tbsp. of dill (chopped)
- Half cup of soy milk (unsweetened)

Method:

1. Mix the listed ingredients in a medium mixing bowl.
2. If you want the dressing to be thin, add a bit of almond milk. Allow the dressing to sit for a few minutes.
3. Chill the prepared dressing.

Notes:

- You can serve the dressing with any savory snacks, sandwiches, quick-bites, salads, etc.
- You can store the leftover dressing in the fridge for two days.
- You can add some ground nuts for enhancing the flavor.

PART III

Chapter 1: Identifying the Mediterranean Diet

We know that certain diets are associated with better health—this is a simple fact of life. We've seen that entire groups of people live longer based on where they live, and to some degree, a good deal of that has to come from somewhere—it has to come from something like diet or environment. In this case, the diet of the people living in the Mediterranean has been found to be incredibly healthy for people—it has been shown that people who are able to enjoy this diet, who are able to eat fresh food by the sea and enjoy the benefits that it has, are able to be far healthier than those who don't have it. That is great for them—but what is their secret?

It turns out, it's all in the lifestyle. The Mediterranean lifestyle, food, and all, is incredibly healthy for you. Studies have shown that people living in Mediterranean countries such as Greece and Italy have been found to have far less risk of death from coronary disease. Their secret is in the diet. Their diet has been shown to reduce the risk of cardiovascular disease, meaning that it is incredibly healthy, beneficial, and something that the vast majority of people in the world could definitely benefit from.

The Mediterranean diet is recommended by doctors and the World Health Organization as being not only healthy but also sustainable, meaning that it is something that is highly recommended, even by the experts. If you've found that you've struggled with weight loss, heart disease, managing your blood pressure, or anything similar to those problems, then the Mediterranean diet is for you. When you follow this diet, you are able to bring health back to your life and enjoy the foods while doing so. It's perfect if you want to be able to enjoy your diet without having to worry about the impacts that it will have on you.

Defining the Mediterranean Lifestyle

The Mediterranean diet is quite simple. It involves eating traditional foods based on one's location. Typically, in the Mediterranean, that is a diet that is rich in veggies, fruits, whole grains, beans, and features olive oil as the fat of choice. Typically, it involves elements beyond just eating as well. While it is important to have healthy food, it is equally important to recognize that the diet encompasses the lifestyle as well. In particular, you can expect to see a few other rules come into play.

In particular, the Mediterranean diet is unique in the sense that it encourages a glass of red wine every now and then. In fact, the diet is associated with moderate drinking, enjoying red wine several times per week, always responsibly, and in contexts that will be beneficial to the drinker. If you want to be able to enjoy the Mediterranean diet and you are pregnant, or against drinking, you can do that, too—but traditionally, the red wine is included and even encouraged in moderation thanks to the antioxidants within it.

Additionally, on the Mediterranean diet, it is common to share meals with friends and family. This is essential—eating is more than just filling the body, it is nurturing the mind and relationships as well. This also comes with the added benefit of also being able to slow down eating—when you are eating the foods on this diet, you will discover that ultimately, you eat less when you're busy having a riveting conversation with someone. The fact that you are slowed down with your eating means that you will fill up sooner and realize that you didn't have to actually eat the food that you did. This means that you eat less and are, therefore managing your portions better as a result.

Finally, the Mediterranean diet focuses on physical activity. Traditionally, you would have had to go out to get the foods that you would eat each day, and that would mean that you'd need to get up, fish, garden, farm, or otherwise prepare your food. Eating locally is still a major component of this diet, as is getting up and being active. You need at least 30 minutes of activity, moderate or mild, per day. Even just walking for half an hour is better than nothing!

The Rules of the Mediterranean Diet

To eat the Mediterranean way, there are a few key factors that can guide you. If you know what you are doing, you can eat well without having to sacrifice flavor for health, and that matters immensely. When you look at the Mediterranean diet closely, you see that there are several tips that will help you to recognize what you need to do to stick to your diet.

Eating fruits and veggies

First, make sure that the bulk of your calories come from fruits and vegetables. You should be eating between 7 and 10 servings of fresh fruits and vegetables every single day—meaning that the bulk of your calories will come from there. Try to stick to locally grown foods that are fresh and in-season—they will have the highest nutritional value.

Reach for the whole grains

Yes, pasta is a major part of the diet in the Mediterranean, and you don't have to give that up entirely—but make sure that any grains that you are enjoying are whole-wheat. This allows you to enjoy foods that are high in fiber and are able to be digested differently than when you use refined carbs instead. While the refined carbs may give you instantaneous energy, they are also not nearly as good for you as whole wheat.

Using healthy fats

When it comes to flavoring or cooking your foods, you need to reach for the healthy fats first. This means choosing out foods that are cooked with olive oil instead of butter or dipping food in olive oil instead of butter. Olive oil, despite being a fat, has not been found to lead to weight gain when used in moderation. It is an incredibly healthy substitute for butter that is loaded up with all sorts of beneficial, heart-healthy antioxidants that will help your cardiovascular system.

Aim for seafood

When it comes to protein, fish, especially fresh fish, is the best choice. Fish should be consumed at least twice per week, and it should be fresh rather than frozen whenever possible. In particular, it is commonly recommended that you reach for salmon or trout, or other fatty fish because the omega-3 fatty acids within them are incredibly healthy for you, and they will serve you well. Even better, if you grill your fish, you have little cleanup.

Reduce red meat

In addition to adding more seafood to your diet, you need to cut out the red meat. The red meats in your diet are no good for you—they have been linked to inflammation that can make it harder for your cardiovascular system.

Enjoy dairy in moderation

When you are on this diet, dairy is not out of the picture entirely. While you should avoid butter, for the most part, it is a good idea for you to enjoy some low-fat Greek yogurt on occasion and add in some cheese to your diet. It is a good thing for you to enjoy these foods to ensure that you have plenty of calcium to keep your body strong.

Spices, not salt

Perhaps one of the most profound differences between most other diets and the Mediterranean diet is the lack of salt. The Mediterranean diet reaches for herbs and spices before adding in salt, meaning that you will be consuming less of it over time. Even better, you will grow to love your new foods without needing salt.

Chapter 2: Savory Mediterranean Meals

Mediterranean Feta Mac and Cheese

Ingredients

- Egg (1, beaten)
- Feta cheese (8 oz., crumbles)
- Macaroni (0.5 lb., whole-wheat)
- Olive oil (3 Tbsp.)
- Salt and pepper to taste
- Sour cream (8 oz.)

Instructions

1. Cook pasta to instructions to create al dente pasta. Drain and place pasta into baking dish. Toss in feta and oil and mix well.
2. Combine your egg and sour cream with salt and pepper. Then mix well and toss over macaroni. Combine and bake at 350F for 30 minutes.

Chickpea Stew

Ingredients

- Bay leaf (1)
- Dry chickpeas (1 c., soaked overnight and peeled)
- Garlic (1 clove, cut in half)
- Lemon to serve
- Olive oil (0.25 c.)
- Onion (1, diced)
- Salt and pepper to taste

Instructions

1. Cover chickpeas in pot with just enough water to cover them and wait to boil. Then rinse and set into clean pot. Toss in all other ingredients but the lemon with just enough water to cover nearly one inch above the beans. Simmer for 2-3 hours and serve with lemons.

Savory Mediterranean Breakfast Muffins

Ingredients

Dry ingredients

- Baking powder (1.5 tsp)
- Baking soda (0.5 tsp)
- Flour (2 c.)
- Salt (0.5 tsp)

Wet ingredients

- Egg (1 large)
- Garlic (1 clove, minced)
- Milk (1 c.)
- Sour cream (0.25 c.)
- Vegetable oil (0.25 c.)

Fillings

- Cheddar cheese (2 c., shredded)
- Feta (2.5 oz., crumbled)
- Green olives (diced, 0.5 c.)
- Green onions (0.5 c., chopped)
- Roasted red peppers (0.5 c., chopped)
- Sun dried tomatoes (diced, 0.5 c.)

Instructions

1. Combine dry ingredients in a bowl. Mix wet ingredients in separate bowl. Combine the two together and mix.
2. Toss in fillings in as few stirs as possible.
3. Place in greased or lined muffin pan, dividing to all 12 recesses.
4. Bake for 25 minutes until golden-brown and crusty at 350F.
5. Cool for 10 minutes and serve warm.

Mediterranean Breakfast Bake

Ingredients

- Artichoke hearts (14-oz. can, drained)
- Bread (6 slices whole-wheat, chopped)
- Eggs (8)
- Feta cheese (0.5 c.)
- Italian sausage (turkey or chicken—1 lb., casings removed)
- Milk (1 c.)
- Olive oil (2 Tbsp., divided)
- Onion (1, chopped)
- Spinach (5 oz.)
- Sun dried tomato (1 c., chopped)

Instructions

1. Warm 1 Tbsp. of your olive oil on moderately high heat. Cook sausage for 8 minutes until it has browned, breaking it up as it cooks. Place it in a dish when it is done.
2. Toss in additional oil, then cook onion until soft, roughly 5 minutes. Toss in spinach until wilting (1 minute).
3. Combine eggs and mix in milk, bread, tomatoes, cheese, artichokes, sausage, and finally, the spinach mix.
4. Place everything in a 2.5 quart baking dish. Let sit for an hour in fridge, or leave overnight.
5. Let casserole sit for 30 minutes after removing from fridge. Then, bake for 45 minutes at 350F until brown. Let rest 10 minutes, then serve.

Mediterranean Pastry Pinwheels

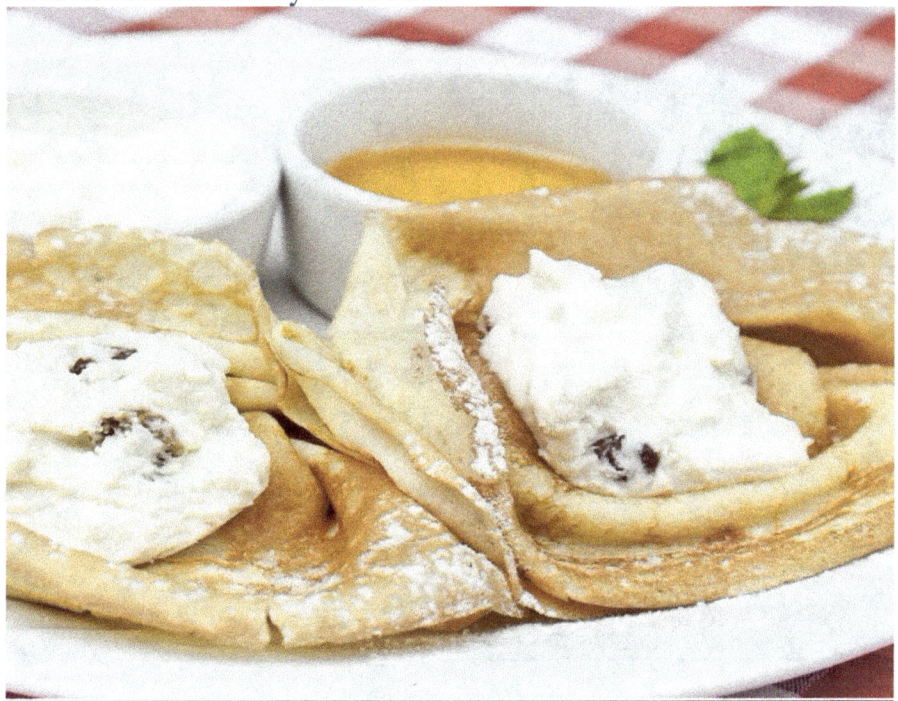

Ingredients

- Cream cheese (8-ounce package, softened)
- Pesto (0.25 c.)
- Provolone cheese (0.75 c.)
- Sun-dried tomatoes (0.5 c., chopped)
- Ripe olives (0.5 c., chopped)
-

Instructions

1. Unroll pastry and trim it up to create 10-inch square.
2. Mix together your cream cheese and pesto until well-combined. Then, mix in other ingredients until combined. Place mixture in even layer across pastry, up to 0.5-inch of edges. Roll and freeze for 30 minutes.
3. Cut whole roll into 16 pieces.
4. Bake at 400F until golden, roughly 15 minutes. Serve.

Chapter 3: Sweet Treats on the Mediterranean Diet

Greek Yogurt Parfait

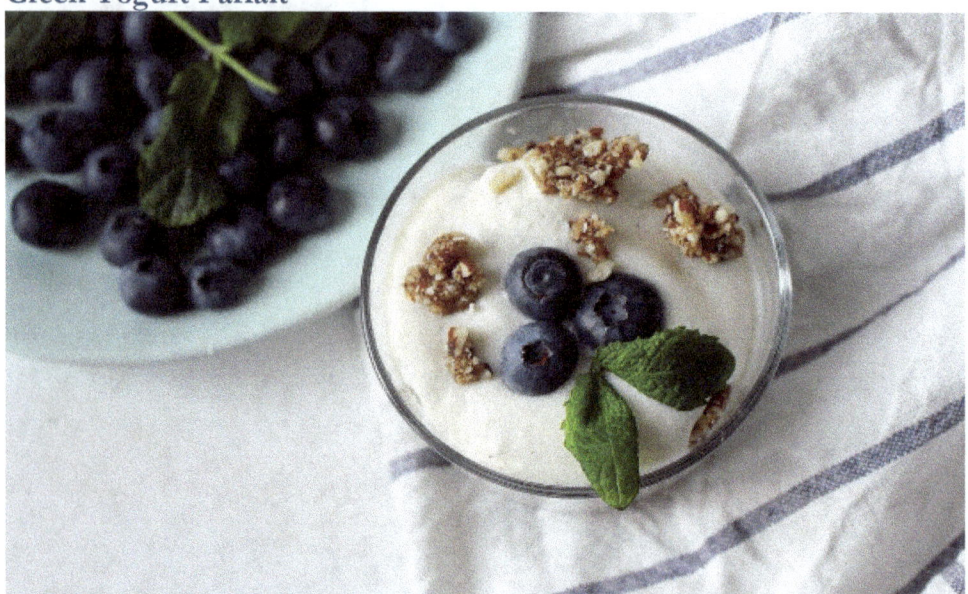

Ingredients

- Almond butter (2 Tbsp.)
- Fresh fruit (1 Tbsp.)
- Greek Yogurt (1 c.)

Instructions

1. Mix together yogurt and 1 Tbsp. of almond butter and put in a bowl. Top with fruit.
2. Warm remaining butter in microwave for 10 minutes, then drizzle atop yogurt. Serve. You can add different toppings to change up the flavor as well.

Overnight Oats

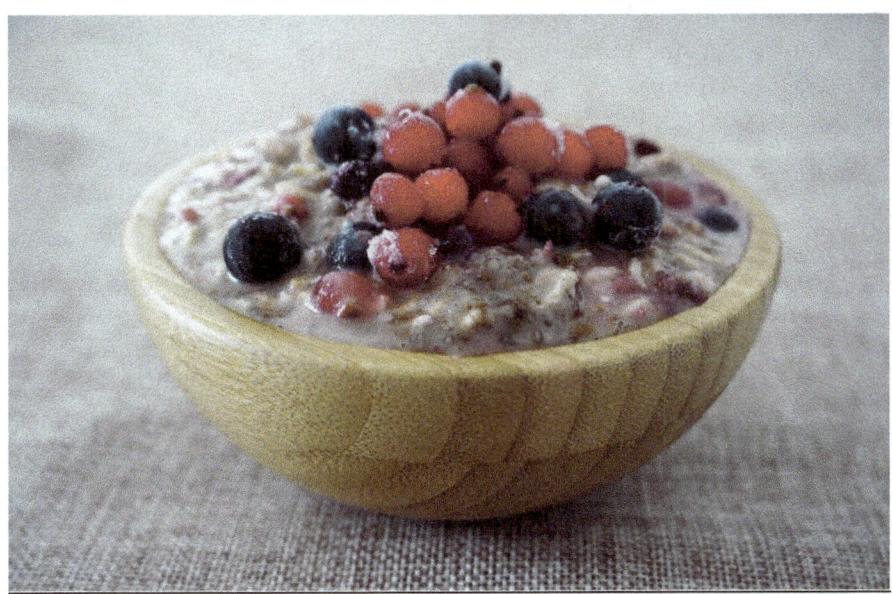

Ingredients

- Chia seeds (1 Tbsp.)
- Greek yogurt (0.25 c.)
- Honey (1 Tbsp.)
- Milk of choice (0.5 c.)
- Old fashioned whole oats (0.5 c.)
- Vanilla extract (0.25 tsp)

Instructions

1. Mix all ingredients into a glass container and leave in fridge for at least 2 hours but preferably overnight. Serve with berries of choice or other desired toppings.

Apple Whipped Yogurt

Ingredients

- Greek yogurt (1 c.)

- Heavy cream (0.5 c.)
- Honey (1 Tbsp.)
- Unsalted butter (2 Tbsp.)
- Apples (2, cored and chopped into small bits)
- Sugar (2 Tbsp.)
- Cinnamon (1/8 tsp)
- Walnut halves (0.25 c., chopped)

Instructions

1. Using a hand mixer, mix together yogurt, honey, and honey until it creates peaks.
2. Heat up your butter in a skillet over a moderate temperature. Cook apples and 1 Tbsp. sugar in pan. Stir and cook for 6-8 minutes until soft. Then, top with the rest of sugar and cinnamon, stirring and cooking an additional 3 minutes. Take it off of the burner and let it rest for 5 minutes.
3. Serve with whipped yogurt in bowl topped with apple, then sprinkle on walnuts.

Chapter 4: Gourmet Meals on the Mediterranean Diet

Garlic-Roasted Salmon and Brussels Sprouts

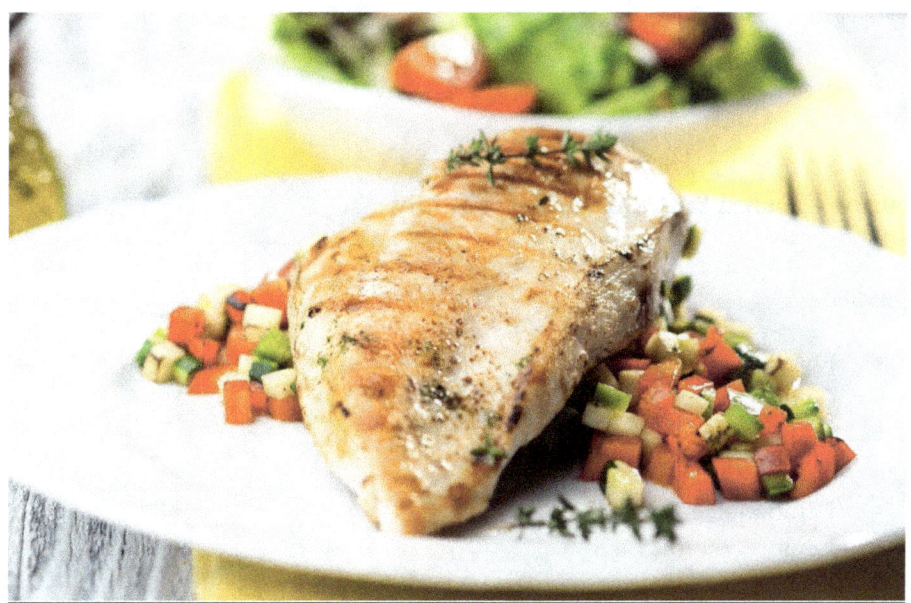

Ingredients

- Brussels sprouts (6 c., trimmed and halved)
- Chardonnay (0.75 c.)
- Garlic cloves (14 large)
- Olive oil (0.25 c.)
- Oregano (2 Tbsp., fresh)
- Pepper (0.75 tsp)
- Salmon fillet (2 lbs., skin-off—cut in 6 pieces)
- Salt (1 tsp)
- Lemon wedges to serve

Instructions

1. Take two cloves of garlic and mince, combining them with oil, 1 Tbsp. of oregano, half of the salt and 1/3 of the pepper. Cut remaining cloves of garlic in halves and toss them with the sprouts. Take 3 Tbsp. of your

garlic oil and toss it with the sprouts in roasting pan. Roast for 15 minutes at 450F.
2. Add wine to the remainder of the oil mixture. Then, remove it from the pan, stir veggies, and place salmon atop it all. Pour the wine mix atop it and season with remaining oregano and salt and pepper. Bake 5-10 minutes until salmon is done. Serve alongside the wedged lemon.

Walnut Crusted Salmon with Rosemary

Ingredients

- Dijon mustard (2 tsp)
- Garlic (1 clove, minced)
- Honey (0.5 tsp)
- Kosher salt (0.5 tsp)
- Lemon juice (1 tsp)
- Lemon zest (0.25 tsp.)
- Olive oil (1 tsp)
- Olive oil spray
- Panko (3 Tbsp.)
- Red pepper (0.25 tsp)
- Rosemary (1 tsp, chopped)
- Salmon (1 pound, skin removed)
- Walnuts (3 Tbsp., finely chopped)
- Parsley and lemon to garnish

Instructions

1. Mix together the mustard, lemon zest and juice, honey, salt and red pepper, and rosemary. In a separate dish, combine the panko with oil and walnuts.
2. Spread mustard across salmon and top with panko mixture. Spray fillets with cooking spray.
3. Cook until fish begins to flake at 425F, roughly 8-10 minutes. Serve with lemon and parsley.

Spaghetti and Clams

Ingredients

- Clams (6.5 lbs.)
- Olive oil (6 Tbsp.)
- White wine (0.5 c.)
- Garlic (3 cloves, sliced)
- Chiles (3, small and crumbled)
- Spaghetti (1 lb.)
- Parsley (3 Tbsp., chopped)
- Salt and pepper to personal preference

Instructions

1. Prepare clams, soaking in clean water and brushing to remove all sand.
2. Warm 2 Tbsp. of oil in large pot. Then, toss in 0.25 c. wine, 1 of the cloves of garlic, and 1 chile. Cook half of the plans at high heat with regular shaking until clams are opened. Remove opened clams and their juices to a larger bowl. Repeat process with second half of clams. Discard any that do not open.
3. Prepare pasta according to packaging to create al dente pasta. Reserve 1 c. pasta water.
4. Warm remainder of oil (2 Tbsp.) in pot over moderate heat, tossing in remainder of garlic and chile. Cook until fragrant, then place all clams and their juices into the pot, tossing to coat well. Then, toss in pasta, mixing well to combine. If necessary, add in cooking liquid. Serve and season with salt/pepper to personal preference with parsley atop.

Braised Lamb and Fennel

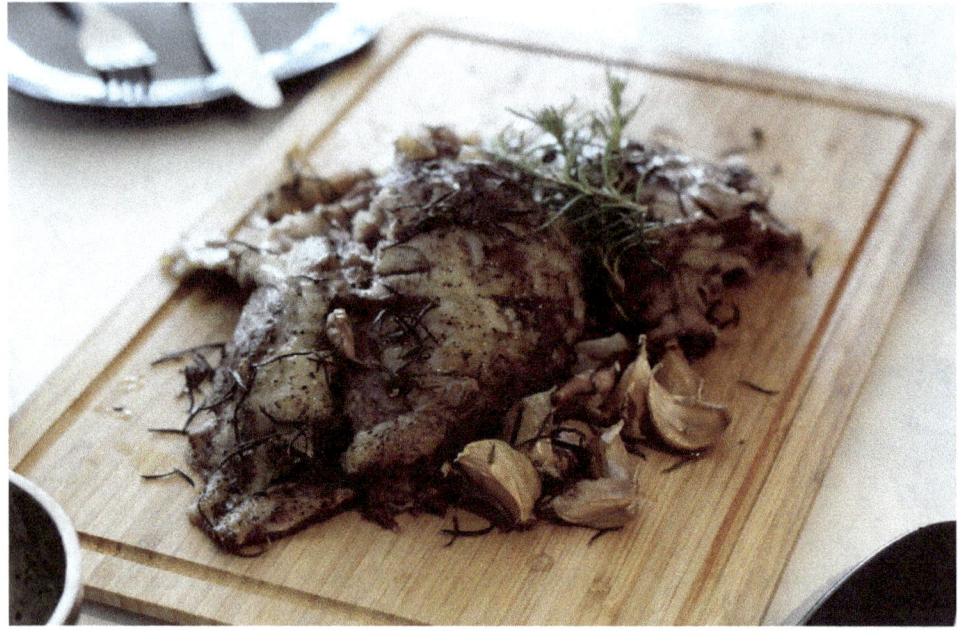

Ingredients

- Bay leaves (2)
- Chicken broth (3 c.)
- Cinnamon stick (1)
- Fennel (1 bulb, chopped)
- Garlic head (chopped in half)
- Lamb shoulder (3 lbs., cut into 8 pieces)
- Olive oil (2 Tbsp.)
- Onion (1, chopped
- Orange (1 with peel, cut into wedges)
- White wine (1 c.)
- Whole peeled tomatoes (14.5 oz. can)

Instructions

1. Dry lamb and season with salt and pepper to taste. Warm oil inside a Dutch oven, and sear lamb on all sides, roughly 6 minutes each side. Move lamb to plate.
2. Place fennel, garlic, and onion in the pot and cook, until browning, roughly 8 minutes. Mix in wine and boil, deglazing the pan. Reduce heat and simmer until it has reduced 50%.
3. Toss in orange, bay leaves, tomatoes, broth, and cinnamon, plus the lamb. Simmer, then cover pot and transfer to oven set to 325F. braise for 1.5-2 hours. Remove lamb and place on clean plate.
4. Strain liquid left in pot, then return it to the pot to boil until thick, roughly 30 minutes.
5. Return lamb to pot to warm. Serve.

Mediterranean Cod

Ingredients

- Black olives (0.66 c., sliced)
- Cod (4 fillets, skinless)
- Fennel seeds (1 tsp)
- Lemon (1, sliced)
- Lemon (juice of ½ lemon)
- Olive oil (6 Tbsp.)
- Onion (1, sliced)
- Parsley (1 Tbsp., chopped)
- Salt and pepper to personal preference
- Tomatoes (0.66 c., diced)

Instructions

1. Warm olive oil at a moderate temperature, sautéing the onion with a pinch of salt until translucent, roughly 10 minutes.
2. Mix in tomato and olives, tossing in the juice as well. Allow it to simmer gently for roughly 5 minutes. Toss in fennel seeds and set aside.
3. Warm the rest of the oil in another pan and fry up the cod for 10 minutes, flipping halfway through until done.
4. Toss tomato sauce over heat to warm, then mix together the parsley, and serve atop the cod with a lemon slice.

Baked Feta with Olive Tapenade

Ingredients

- Baked pita or crusty bread to serve
- Feta cheese (6 oz.)
- Garlic (2 cloves)
- Green olives (0.33 c., sliced)
- Harissa paste (3 Tbsp.)
- Olive oil (3 Tbsp.)
- Parsley (3 Tbsp., fresh chopped)
- Roasted red peppers (16-oz. jar, drained)
- Salt (0.75 tsp.)
- Tomato paste (2 Tbsp.)
- Walnuts (0.5 c., halved)

Instructions

1. In a blender, combine your peppers, 0.25 c. walnuts, harissa and tomato paste, garlic, and 0.5 tsp of your salt until mostly consistent. It doesn't have to be perfect, but should be well combined.
2. Take half of mixture into baking dish that has been sprayed with cooking spray. Top with half of your feta, then spoon the rest of the red pepper sauce atop it.
3. Top with the last of the feta and bake until bubbly, roughly 25 minutes. Broil for the last 2.
4. While that bakes, make your tapenade. This requires you to combine your remaining ingredients together.
5. Remove mixture from oven and top with tapenade. Serve immediately with crusty bread or pita chips.

Chapter 5: 30-Minutes or Less Meals
Vegetarian Toss Together Mediterranean Pasta Salad

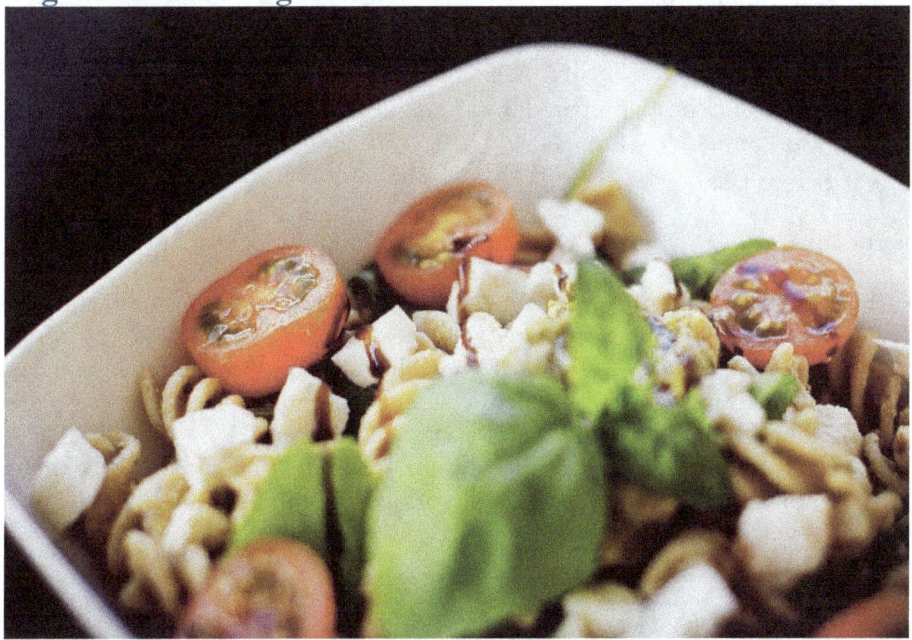

Ingredients

- Artichoke hearts (12 oz. jar, drained)
- Balsamic vinegar (2 Tbsp.)
- Kalamata olives (12-ounce jar, drained and chopped)
- Olive oil (2 Tbsp.)
- Pasta (8 oz., wheat)
- Salt to personal preference
- Sun-dried tomatoes in oil (1.5 oz. jar, drained)

Instructions

1. Prepare pasta according to packaging.
2. Mix together olives, tomatoes, and artichoke.
3. Drain pasta and add them to a bowl with artichoke mixture. Then, top with vinegar and olive oil, mix well, and serve warm.

Vegetarian Aglio e Olio and Broccoli

Ingredients

- Olive oil (3 Tbsp.)
- Cayenne peppers (3)
- Garlic (3 cloves, sliced)
- Broccoli (1 head, prepared in florets)
- Spaghetti (7 oz. whole wheat)
- Salt to taste

Instructions

1. Boil water and prepare spaghetti according to instructions until al dente. Drain and reserve.
2. In a pan, heat up 1 Tbsp. of your olive oil at a moderate temperature, then toss in the garlic and peppers, sautéing until fragrant. Remove garlic from heat and set aside.
3. Toss broccoli into pan and cook for 4 minutes. Then toss in spaghetti, garlic, and remaining oil. Cook for an additional minute or two, then serve.

Cilantro and Garlic Baked Salmon

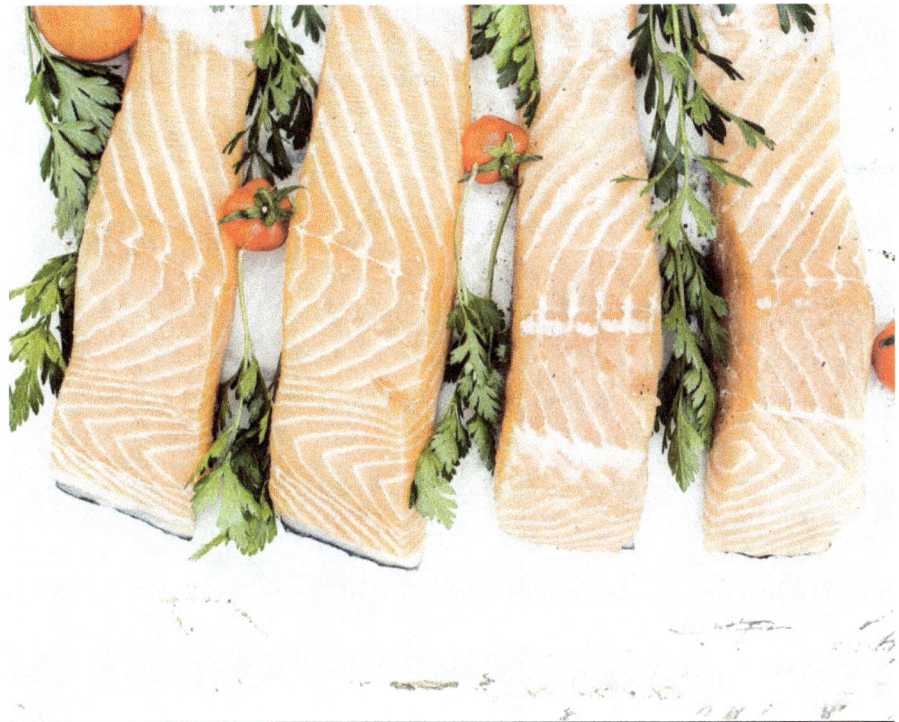

Ingredients

- Cilantro (stems trimmed)
- Garlic (4 cloves, chopped)
- Lime (0.5, cut into rounds)
- Lime juice (1 lime's worth)
- Olive oil (0.5 c.)
- Salmon fillet (2 pounds, skin removed)
- Salt to taste
- Tomato (cut into rounds)

Instructions

1. Allow salmon to come to room temp for 20 minutes while oven preheats to a temperature of 425 F.
2. While you wait, take a processor and combine garlic, cilantro, lime juice, and olive oil with a pinch of salt. Combine well.

3. Place fillet into baking pan that has been greased. Top with a light sprinkle of salt and pepper. Then spread cilantro sauce atop fillet, coating whole salmon. Top with tomato and lime.
4. Bake for 6 minutes per 0.5 inch of thickness (1-inch fillets take around 8-10 minutes). Let rest for 5-10 minutes out of the oven. Serve.

Harissa Pasta

Ingredients

- Pasta (2 cups)
- Red bell pepper (1)
- Red onion (1)
- Pine nuts (2 Tbsp.)
- Harissa paste (2 Tbsp.)

Instructions

1. Roast onions and peppers with olive oil at 400F for 20 minutes. Remove from oven and dice.
2. Prepare pasta to instructions on package. While pasta cooks, toast your pine nuts until browned in frying pan.
3. Drain pasta, leaving a touch of the water. Then, add in diced roasted veggies and harissa. Serve topped with pine nuts.

Chapter 6: 1-Hour-or-Less Meals

1 Hour Baked Cod

Ingredients

- Basil (0.5 tsp., dried)
- Bay leaf (1)
- Capers (1 small jar)
- Cod fillets (2 pounds)
- Fennel seeds (1 tsp., crushed)
- Garlic (1 clove, minced)
- Lemon juice (0.25 c., fresh)
- Olive oil (2 tsp)
- Onion (1, sliced)
- Orange juice (o.25 c., fresh)
- Orange peel (1 Tbsp.)
- Oregano (0.5 tsp., dried)
- Salt and pepper to personal preference
- White wine (1 c., dry)
- Whole tomatoes (16-oz. can, chopped and reserving juice)

Instructions

1. Warm oven to 375F.
2. In cast iron skillet, warm oil. Then, sauté your onion for 5 minutes. At this point, mix in all other ingredients but fish. Allow to simmer for 30 minutes.
3. Place fillets into skillet and top with most of the sauce. Allow to bake for 15 minutes until fish flakes.

Grilled Chicken Mediterranean Salad

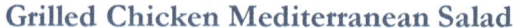

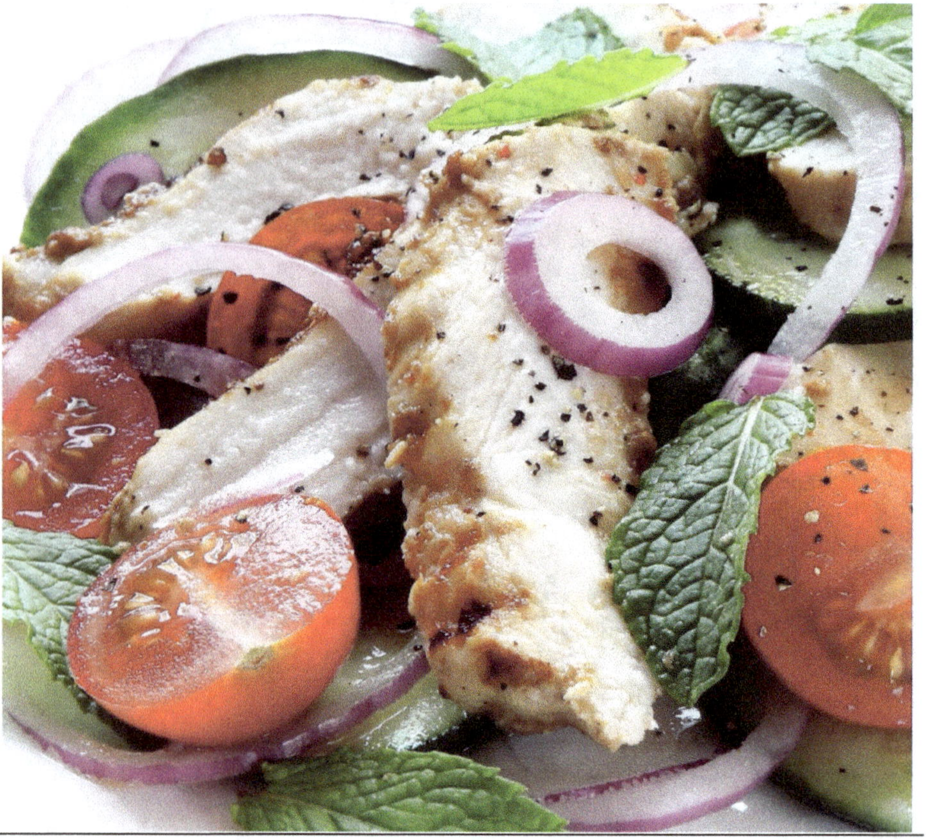

Ingredients

- Artichoke hearts (0.33 c., chopped)
- Balsamic vinegar (2 Tbsp.)
- Basil (1 tsp, dried)
- Chicken breasts (3, cut into bite-sized chunks)
- Cucumber (0.75 c., diced)
- Feta cheese (0.25 c.)
- Garlic (1 clove, minced)
- Greek yogurt (2 Tbsp.)
- Green onions (0.25 c., chopped)
- Kalamata olives (3 Tbsp., sliced)
- Kosher salt (0.5 tsp)
- Lemon juice (3 Tbsp + 1 tsp.)

- Olive oil (3 Tbsp. + 2 Tbsp.)
- Onion powder (0.5 tsp)
- Parsley (0.5 tsp)
- Pesto (4 tsp)
- Pinch of red pepper
- Roasted red pepper (6 Tbsp., sliced)
- Romaine (4 c., chopped)
- Shiitake mushrooms
- Spinach (4 c., chopped)
- Tomato (0.75 c., diced)
- White wine vinegar (4 tsp)

Instructions

1. Create your salad. Each plate should have a bed of romaine and spinach, topped with cucumber, tomato, artichoke, peppers, olives, and cheese.
2. Combine your tsp of lemon juice, wine vinegar, and pesto in a jar and shake to combine. Then, add in yogurt and 2 Tbsp. oil, mixing well until well-incorporated.
3. Prepare your chicken. Let it marinade in a mixture of 3 Tbsp. lemon juice, balsamic vinegar, remaining oil, and all seasonings for at least 30 minutes. Soak some wooden skewers in water during this time.
4. Make kebabs out of chicken and mushroom, alternating bite of chicken and bite of mushroom until chicken is gone. Grill for 10 to 15 minutes until done.
5. Drizzle salad with the vinaigrette, then place a kebab atop each. Serve.

Lemon Herb Chicken and Potatoes One Pot Meal

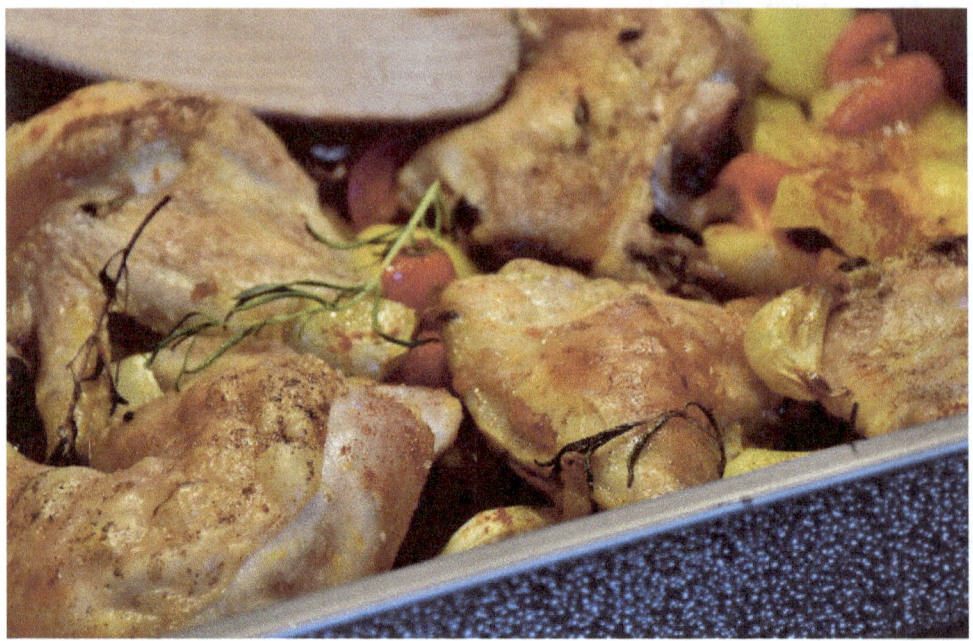

Ingredients

- Baby potatoes (8, halved)
- Basil (3 tsp, dried)
- Bell pepper (1, seeds removed and wedged)
- Chicken thighs (4, skin and bone on)
- Garlic (4 large cloves, crushed)
- Kalamata olives (4 Tbsp., pitted)
- Lemon juice (1 lemon's worth)
- Olive oil (3 Tbsp.)
- Oregano (2 tsp, dried)
- Parsley (2 tsp, dried)
- Red onion (wedged)
- Red wine vinegar (1 Tbsp.)
- Salt (2 tsp)
- Zucchini (1 large, sliced)

- Lemons for garnish

Instructions

1. Combine juice from lemon, 2 Tbsp. olive oil, vinegar, seasonings, and garlic into dish. Pour half to reserve for later, then place chicken in half. Let sit for 15 minutes (or overnight if you would like to prep the day before)
2. Warm oven to 430F. Sear chicken in cast iron skillet in remaining olive oil, about 4 minutes per side. Drain all but 1 Tbsp. of fat.
3. Place all veggies around the thighs. Top with remaining marinade and combine well to cover everything.
4. Cover pan and bake for 35 minutes until soft and chicken is to temperature. Then, broil for 5 minutes or until golden brown. Top with olives and lemon to serve.

Vegetarian Mediterranean Quiche

Ingredients

- Butter (2 Tbsp.)
- Cheddar cheese (1 c., shredded)
- Eggs (4 large)
- Feta (0.33 c.)
- Garlic (2 cloves, minced)
- Kalamata olives (0.25 c., sliced)
- Milk (1.25 c.)
- Onion (1, diced)
- Oregano (1 tsp, dried)
- Parsley (1 tsp, dried)
- Pie crust (1, prepared)
- Red pepper (1, diced)
- Salt and pepper to personal preference
- Spinach (2 c., fresh)
- Sun dried tomatoes (0.5 c.)

Instructions

1. Soak sun-dried tomatoes in boiling water for 5 minutes before draining and chopping.
2. Prepare a pie dish with a crust, fluting the edges.
3. In a skillet, melt your butter, then cook your garlic and onions in it until they become fragrant. Combine in the red peppers for another 3 minutes until softened. Then, toss in your spinach, olives, and seasoning. Cook until the spinach wilts, about 5 minutes. Take it off of the heat and toss in your feta and tomatoes. Then, carefully place mixture into the crust, spreading it into a nice, even layer.
4. Mix milk, eggs, and half of cheddar cheese together. Pour it into the crust. Then, top with cheddar.
5. Bake for 50 minutes at 375 f. until crust is browned and egg is done.

Herbed Lamb and Veggies

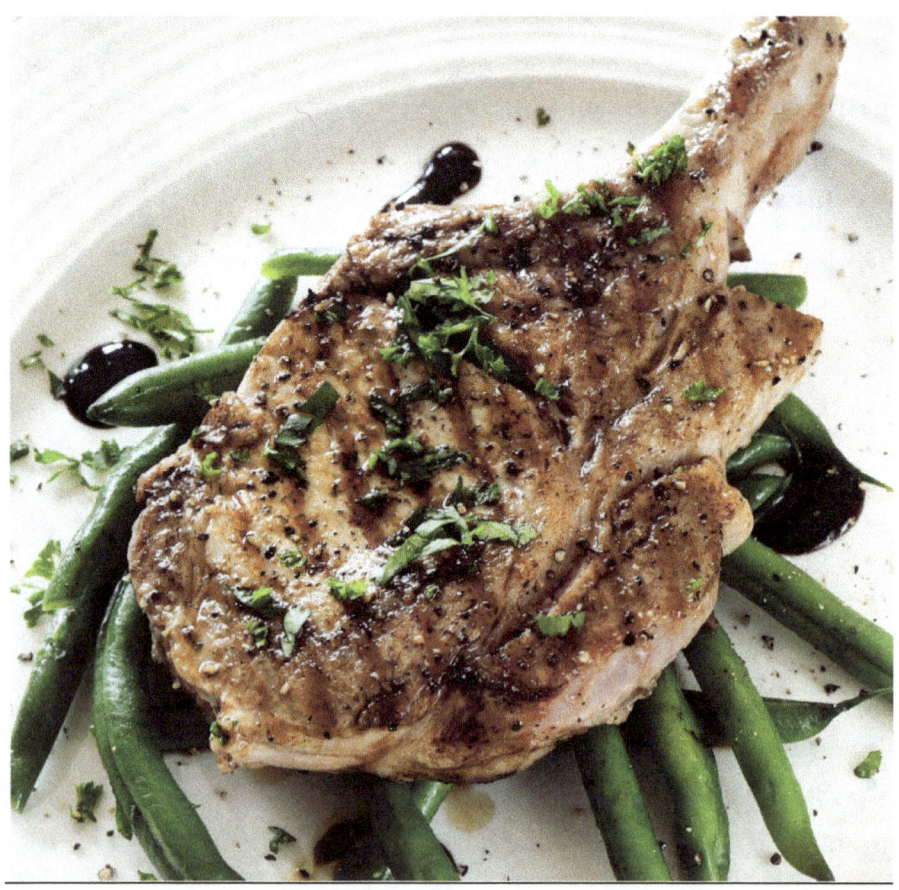

Ingredients

- Bell pepper (2, any color, seeds removed and cut into bite-sized chunks)
- Lamb cutlets (8 lean)
- Mint (2 Tbsp., fresh, chopped)
- Olive oil (1 Tbsp.)
- Red onion (1, wedged)
- Sweet potato (1 large, peeled, and chunked)
- Thyme (1 Tbsp., fresh, chopped)
- Zucchini (2, chunked)

Instructions

1. Assemble your veggies onto a baking sheet and coat with oil and black pepper. Bake at 400F for 25 minutes.
2. As veggies bake, trim fat from the lamb. Then, combine the herbs with a bit of freshly ground pepper. Coat the lamb in the seasoning.
3. Remove veggies, flip, and push to one side of pan. Then, arrange your cutlets onto the baking pan as well. Bake for 10 minutes, flip, then cook an additional 10 minutes. Combine well, then serve.

Chicken and Couscous Mediterranean Wraps

Ingredients

- Parsley (1 c., fresh and chopped)
- Olive oil (3 Tbsp.)
- Garlic (2 tsp, minced)
- Salt (pinch)
- Pepper (pinch)
- Chicken tenders (1 pound)
- Tomato (1, chopped)
- Cucumber (1, chopped)
- Spinach wraps (4 1o-inch)
- Water (0.5 c)
- Mint (0.5 c., fresh chopped)
- Lemon juice (0.25 c.)
- Couscous (0.33 c.)

Instructions

1. Cook couscous in boiling water according to directions on package.
2. Mix together your lemon juice, oil, garlic, salt and pepper, mint, and parsley.
3. Coat chicken in 1 Tbsp. of your mixture from previous step and top with a pinch of salt. Cook in skillet until completely cooked, usually just a few minutes per side.
4. Wait for chicken to cool, then chop into bites.
5. Pour the remainder of your parsley mixture into the couscous with cucumbers and tomato bits.
6. Place 0.75 c. of couscous mixture into a tortilla, then spread chicken atop it, rolling them up and serving.

Sheet Pan Shrimp

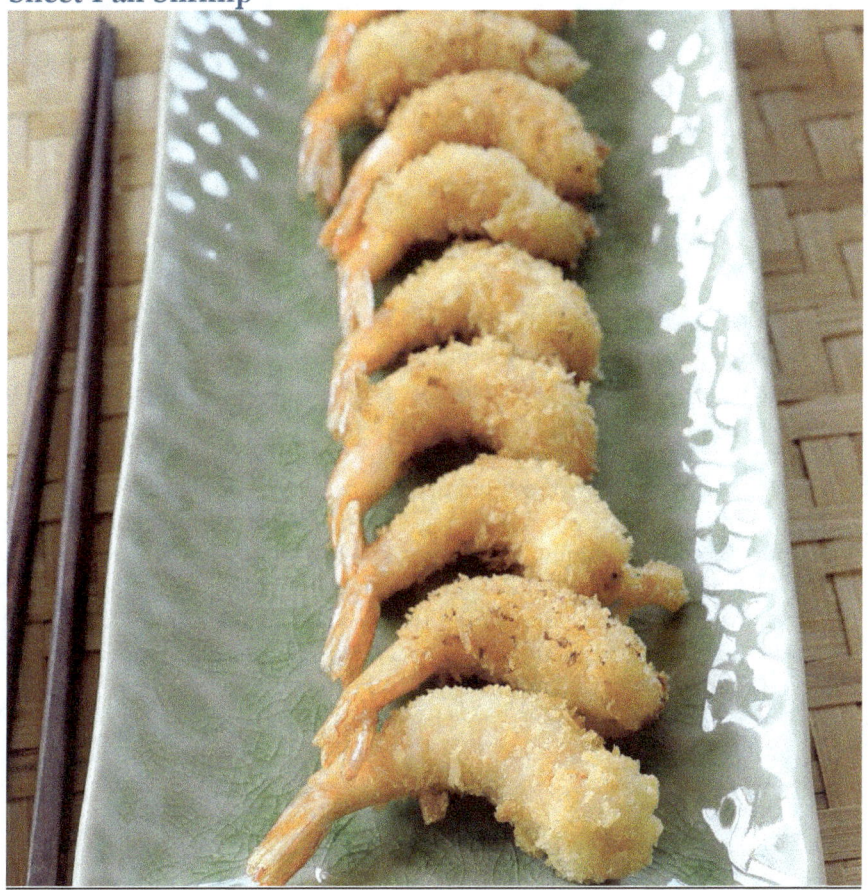

Ingredients

For shrimp

- Feta cheese (0.5 c.)
- Fingerling potatoes (2 c., halved)
- Green beans (6 oz., trimmed)
- Olive oil (3 Tbsp.)
- Pepper (1 tsp)
- Red onion (1 medium, sliced)
- Red pepper (1 medium, sliced)
- Salt (1 tsp)
- Shrimp (1 lb., deveined and peeled)

For Marinade

- Garlic (1 Tbsp., minced)
- Oregano (0.5 tsp)
- Greek yogurt (1 c.)
- Lemon juice (2 Tbsp.)
- Paprika (0.5 tsp)
- Parsley (2 Tbsp., chopped)

Instructions

1. Combine all marinade ingredients and set aside.
2. Take shrimp in a bowl with 0.5 c. of the marinade. Let them sit for 30 minutes.
3. During rest time, set up your baking sheet with foil or parchment, and prepare your veggies. Chop them up and toss onto baking sheet, drizzling them with the olive oil and giving them a quick sprinkle of salt and pepper. Bake for roughly 20 minutes at 400F, then remove from oven. Take out all green beans and set to the side.
4. Place shrimp in one layer across the pan and bake for an additional 10 minutes until shrimp is done. Serve with veggies and shrimp in bowls, topped with 2 Tbsp. feta and a spoonful of yogurt marinade.

Mediterranean Mahi Mahi

Ingredients

- Basil (6 leaves, freshly chopped)
- Capers (4 Tbsp.)
- Garlic (2 cloves, chopped)
- Italian seasoning (pinch)
- Kalamata olives (25, chopped)
- Lemon juice (1 tsp)
- Mahi mahi (1 pound)
- Olive oil (2 Tbsp.)
- Onion (o.5, chopped)
- Parmesan cheese (3 Tbsp.)
- Diced tomatoes (15 oz. can)
- White wine (0.25 c.)

Instructions

1. Warm olive oil in a pan and then cook onions until translucent. Toss in garlic and seasoning and stir to mix well. Then, add in your can of tomatoes, wine, olives, lemon, and roughly half of the chopped basil. Drop heat down and toss in parmesan cheese. Cook until bubbling.
2. Put fish into a baking pan, then top with the sauce. Bake for 20 minutes at 425 F until fish is to temperature.

Chapter 7: Slow Cooker Meals

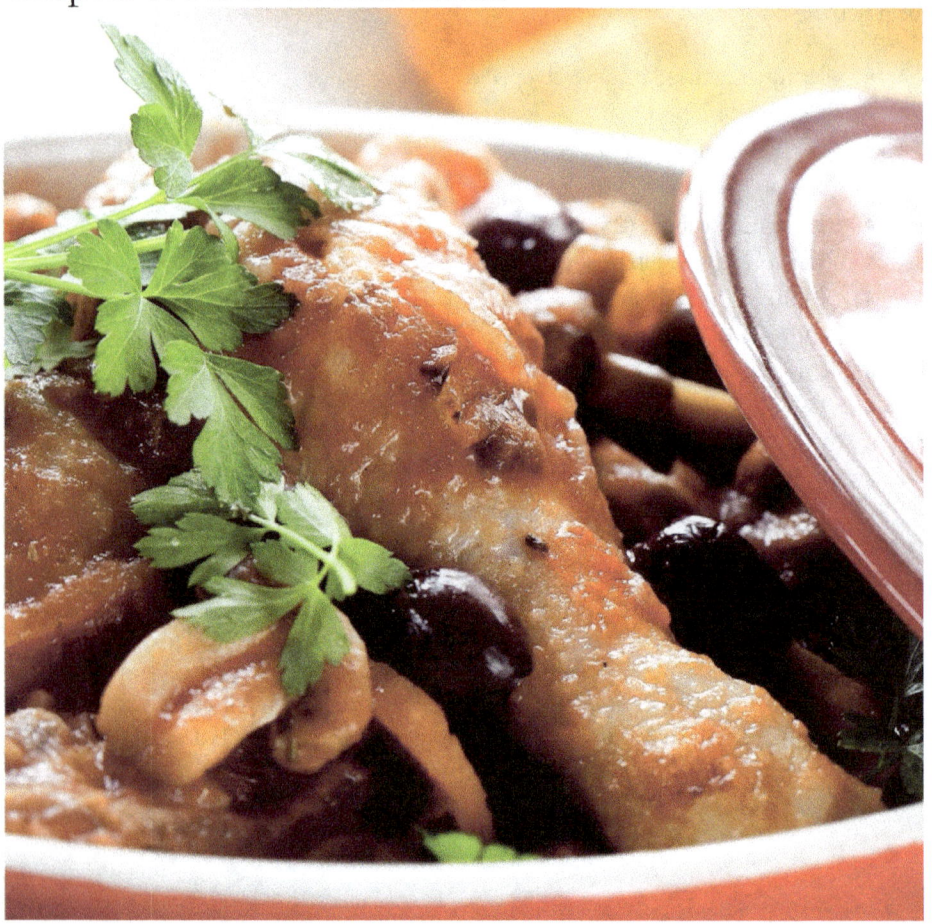

Slow Cooker Mediterranean Chicken

Ingredients

- Bay leaf (1)
- Capers (1 Tbsp.)
- Chicken broth (0.5 c.)
- Chicken thighs (2 pounds, bone and skin removed)
- Garlic (3 cloves, minced)
- Kalamata olives (1 c.)
- Olive oil (1 Tbsp.)
- Oregano (1 tsp)

- Roasted red pepper (1 c.)
- Rosemary (1 tsp, dried)
- Salt and pepper to taste
- Sweet onion (1, thinly sliced)
- Thyme (1 tsp, dried)
- Optional fresh lemon wedges to juice for serving

Instructions

1. Sauté the chicken in olive oil to brown on both sides, then remove it from the pan. Then, sauté the onions and garlic as well until beginning to soften, roughly 5 minutes.
2. Put chicken, onion, garlic, and all other ingredients into a slow cooker and leave it to cook for 4 hours on low. Season to taste.

Slow Cooker Vegetarian Mediterranean Stew

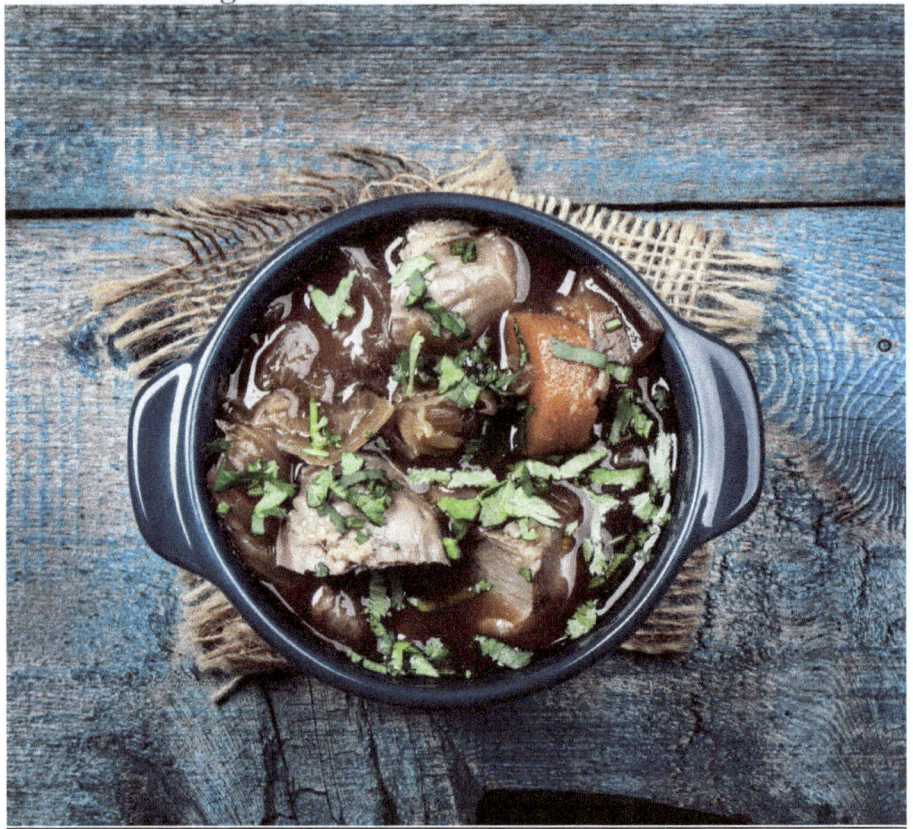

Ingredients

- Carrot (0.75 c., chopped)
- Chickpeas (15 oz. can)
- Crushed red pepper (0.5 tsp)
- Fire-roasted diced tomatoes (2 14-oz. cans)
- Garlic (4 cloves, minced)
- Ground pepper (0.25 tsp)
- Kale (8 c., chopped)
- Lemon juice (1 Tbsp.)
- Olive oil (3 Tbsp.)
- Onion (1, chopped)
- Oregano (1 tsp)
- Salt (0.75 tsp)
- Vegetable broth (3 c.)

- Basil leaves (garnish)
- Lemon wedges (garnish)

Instructions

1. Mix tomatoes, onion, carrot, broth, seasonings, and garlic into the slow cooker. Cook on low for 6 hours.
2. Take out 0.25 c. of the liquid in the slow cooker after 6 hours and transfer it to a bowl. Take out 2 Tbsp. of chickpeas and mash them with the liquid until nice and smooth.
3. Combine mash, kale, juice from lemon, and whole chickpeas. Cook for about 30 minutes, until kale is tender, then serve garnished with the basil leaves and lemon wedges.

Vegetarian Slow Cooker Quinoa

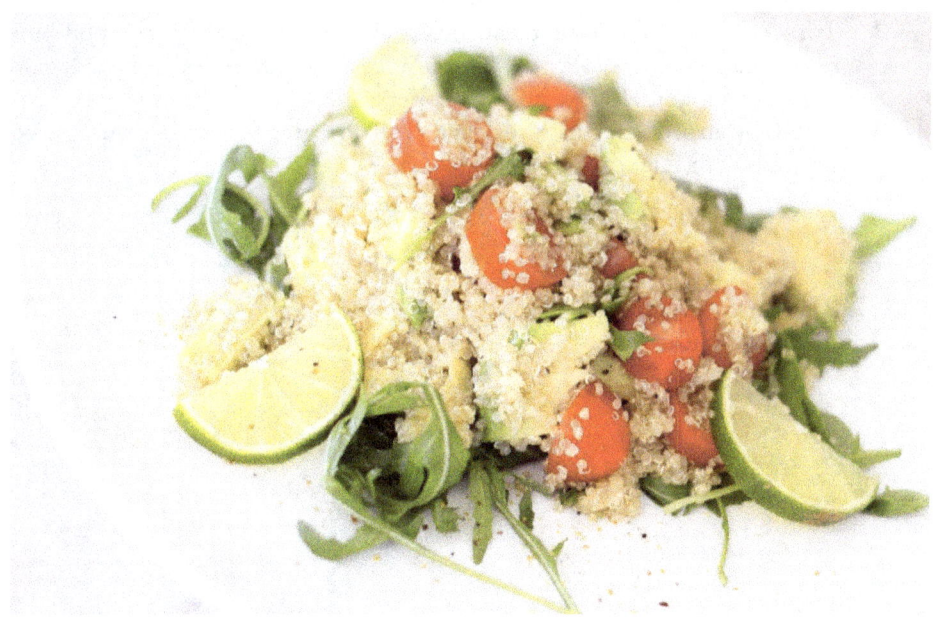

Ingredients

- Arugula (4 c.)
- Chickpeas (1 15.5 oz. can, rinsed and drained)
- Feta cheese (0.5 c)
- Garlic (2 cloves, minced)
- Kalamata olives (12, halved)
- Kosher salt (0.75 tsp)
- Lemon juice (2 tsp)
- Olive oil (2.25 Tbsp.)
- Oregano (2 Tbsp., fresh and coarsely chopped
- Quinoa (1.5 c., uncooked)
- Red onion (1 c., sliced)
- Roasted red pepper (0.5 c., drained and chopped)
- Vegetable stock (2.25 c.)

Instructions

1. Mix your broth with the onion, garlic, quinoa, chickpeas, and 1.5 tsp of olive oil. Sprinkle half of the salt atop it. Mix and cook on low until quinoa is done, roughly 3 or 4 hours.
2. Turn off the slow cooker and mix well. In a separate bowl, combine remaining olive oil, salt, and lemon juice together. Then, mix that into the slow cooker, along with the peppers.
3. Combine in the arugula and leave until the greens start to wilt. Serve, topping with feta, oregano, and olives.

Slow-Cooked Chicken and Chickpea Soup

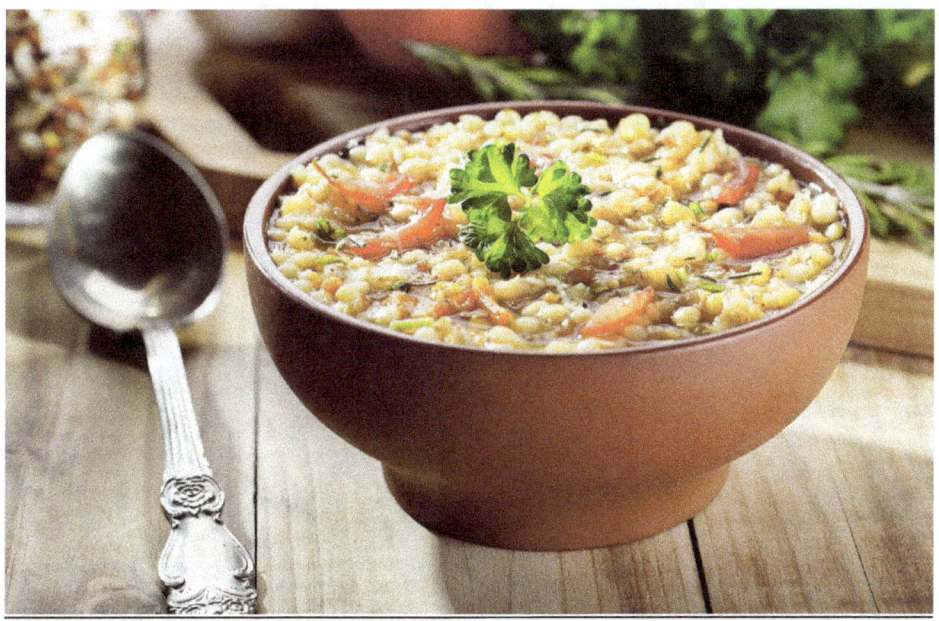

Ingredients

- Artichoke hearts (14 oz. can, drained and chopped)
- Bay leaf (1)
- Cayenne (0.25 tsp)
- Chicken thighs (2 lbs., skins removed)
- Cumin (4 tsp)
- Diced tomatoes (1 15-ounce can)
- Dried chickpeas (1.5 c., allow to soak overnight)
- Garlic cloves (4, chopped)
- Olives (0.25 c., halved)
- Paprika (4 tsp)
- Pepper (0.25 tsp)
- Salt (0.5 tsp)
- Tomato paste (2 Tbsp.)
- Water (4 c.)
- Yellow onion (chopped)
- Parsley or cilantro (garnish)

Instructions

1. Drain your soaked chickpeas and place them into your slow cooker (large preferred). Mix in the water, onions and garlic, tomatoes (undrained), tomato paste, and all seasonings. Combine well, then add in the chicken.
2. Leave it to cook for 8 hours at low, or 4 at high.
3. Remove the chicken and allow it to cool on a cutting board. At the same time, remove the bay leaf, then add in the artichoke and olives. Season with additional salt if necessary to taste. Chop up chicken, removing the bones, and then mix it back into the soup. Serve the soup with the parsley or cilantro garnishing the top.

Slow Cooked Brisket
Ingredients

- Beef broth (0.5 c.)
- Brisket (3 lbs.)
- Cold water (0.25 c.)
- Fennel bulbs (2, cored, trimmed, and cut into wedges)
- Flour
- Italian seasoning (3 tsp)
- Italian seasoning diced tomatoes (14.5 oz. can)
- Lemon peel (1 tsp., fine shreds)
- Olives (0.5 c.)
- Parsley for garnish
- Pepper (pinch)
- Salt (pinch)

Instructions

1. Trim meat, then season with 1 tsp Italian seasoning. Put it in slow cooker with the cut-up fennel on top.
2. Mix together the tomatoes, broth, peel, olives, salt and pepper, and the last of the Italian seasoning.
3. Cook at low for 10 hours, or high for 5.
4. Take meat out of the cooker and reserve all juice. Arrange meat with veggies on a serving platter.
5. Remove fat from top of the juices.
6. Take 2 c. of juices in saucepan. Mix together water and flour, then combine it into the juice. Cook until gravy forms.
7. Serve meat topped with gravy and garnish with parsley

Vegan Bean Soup with Spinach

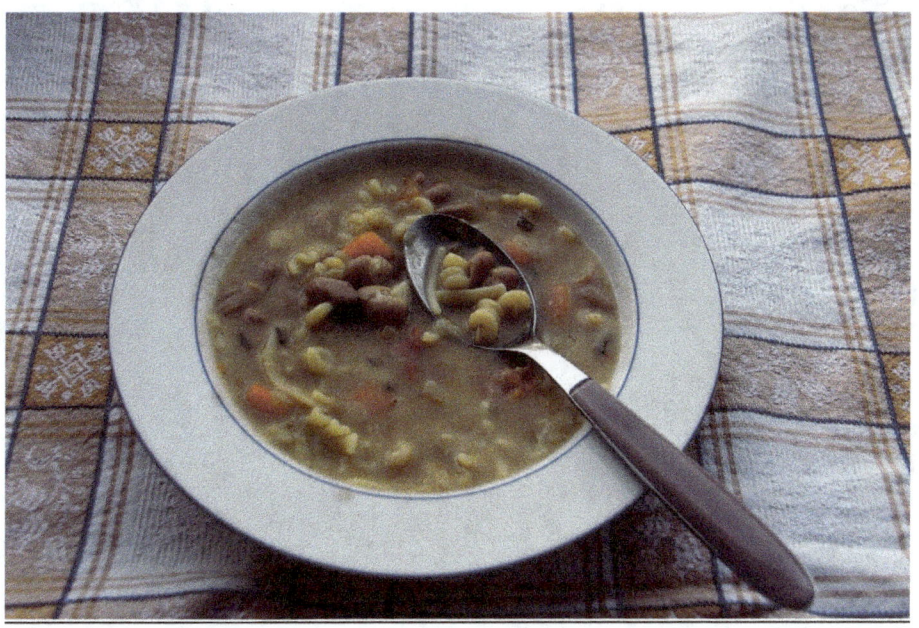

Ingredients

- Vegetable broth (3 14-oz. cans)
- Tomato puree (15 oz. can)
- Great Northern or White beans (15 oz. can)
- White rice (0.5 c)
- Onion (0.5 c., chopped)
- Garlic (2 cloves, minced)
- Basil (1 tsp., dried)
- Pinch of salt
- Pinch of pepper
- Kale or spinach (8 c., chopped)

Instructions

1. Mix everything but leafy greens together in your slow cooker. Cook for 5 or 7 hours on low, or 2.5 hours on high.
2. Toss in leafy greens. Wait for them to wilt and serve.

Moroccan Lentil Soup

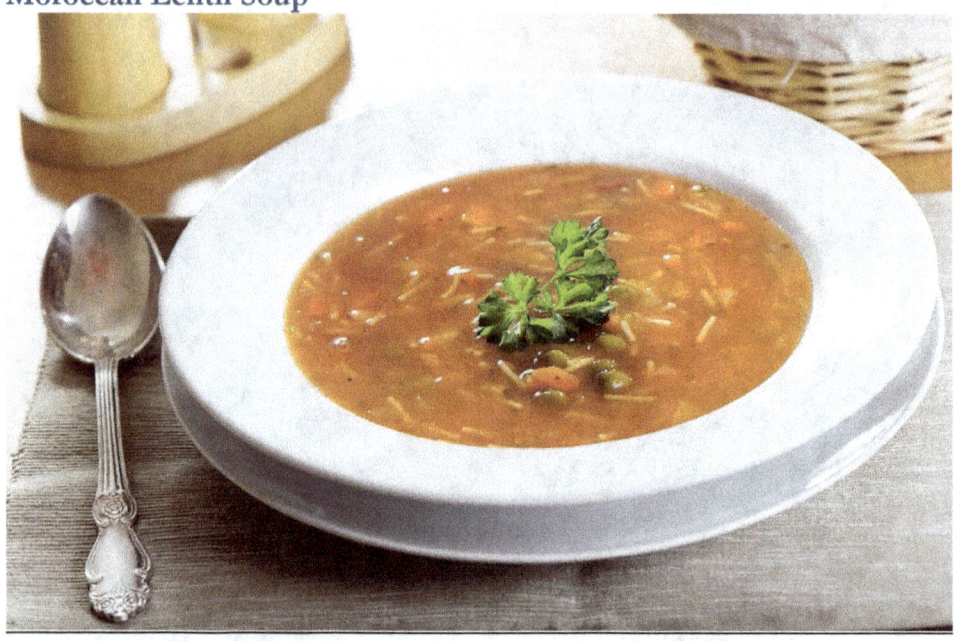

Ingredients

- Carrots (2 c., chopped)
- Cauliflower (3 c.)
- Cinnamon (0.25 tsp)
- Cumin (1 tsp)
- Diced tomato (28 oz.)
- Fresh cilantro (0.5 c.)
- Fresh spinach (4 c.)
- Garlic (4 cloves, minced)
- Ground coriander (1 tsp)
- Lemon juice (2 Tbsp.)
- Lentils (1.75 c.)
- Olive oil (2 tsp)
- Onion (2 c., chopped)
- Pepper (pinch)
- Tomato paste (2 Tbsp.)
- Turmeric (1 tsp)
- Vegetable broth (6 c.)
- Water (2 c.)

Instructions

1. Mix everything but spinach, cilantro, and lemon juice. Cook until lentils soften. This will be 4-5 hours if you use high heat, or 10 hours on low.
2. Mix spinach when just 30 minutes remains on cook time.
3. Just before serving, top with cilantro and lemon juice.

Chapter 8: Vegetarian and Vegan Meals

Vegetarian Greek Stuffed Mushrooms

Ingredients

- Cherry tomatoes (0.5 c., quartered)
- Feta cheese (0.33 c.)
- Garlic (1 clove, mixed)
- Ground pepper (0.5 tsp)
- Kalamata olives (2 Tbsp.)
- Olive oil (3 Tbsp.)
- Oregano (1 Tbsp., fresh and roughly chopped)
- Portobello mushrooms (4, cleaned with stems and gills taken out)
- Salt (0.25 tsp)
- Spinach (1 c., chopped)

Instructions

1. Begin by setting your oven. This recipe requires 400F for baking.
2. Mix together your salt and 0.25 tsp pepper, garlic, and 2 Tbsp. of oil, and use it to cover your mushrooms, inside and out.
3. Set the mushrooms onto your baking pan and allow it to cook for 10 minutes.
4. Mix together your remaining ingredients and combine well. Then, when the mushrooms are done, remove them from the oven and then fill them up with your filling.
5. Allow to cook for another 10 minutes.

Vegetarian Cheesy Artichoke and Spinach Stuffed Squash

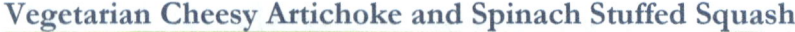

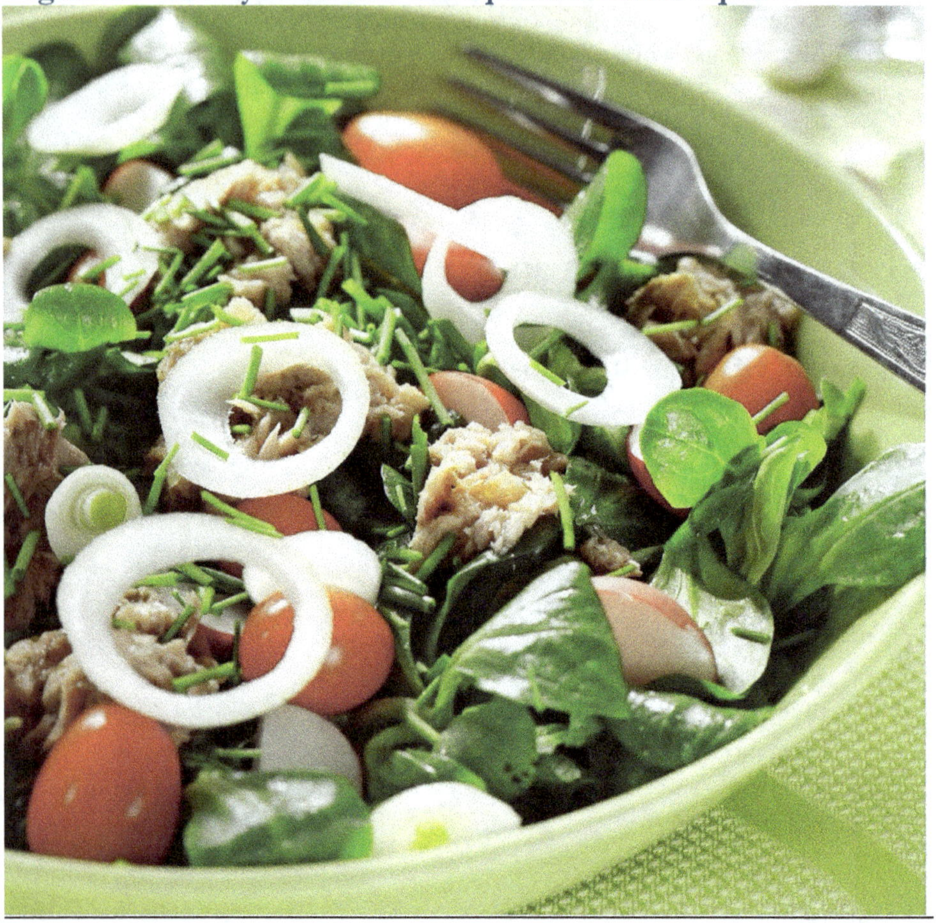

Ingredients

- Artichoke Hearts (10 oz., frozen—thawed and chopped up)
- Baby spinach (5 oz.)
- Cream cheese (4 oz., softened)
- Parmesan cheese (0.5 c.)
- Pepper (pinch to taste)
- Red pepper and basil (for garnish)
- Salt (pinch to taste)
- Spaghetti squash (1, cut in half and cleaned out of seeds)
- Water (3 Tbsp.)

Instructions

1. Microwave your squash, flat side down, with 2 Tbsp. of your water uncovered for 10-15 minutes.
2. Mix together your spinach and water into a skillet until they begin to wilt. Then drain and reserve for later.
3. Preheat your oven set to broil with the rack at the upper 1/3 point.
4. Remove flesh from squash with a fork, then place the shells onto a sheet for the oven. Then stir in your artichoke, cheeses, and a pinch of salt and pepper to the squash flesh. Combine thoroughly, then split it between the two shells. Broil for 3 minutes and top with red pepper and basil to taste.

Vegan Mediterranean Buddha Bowl

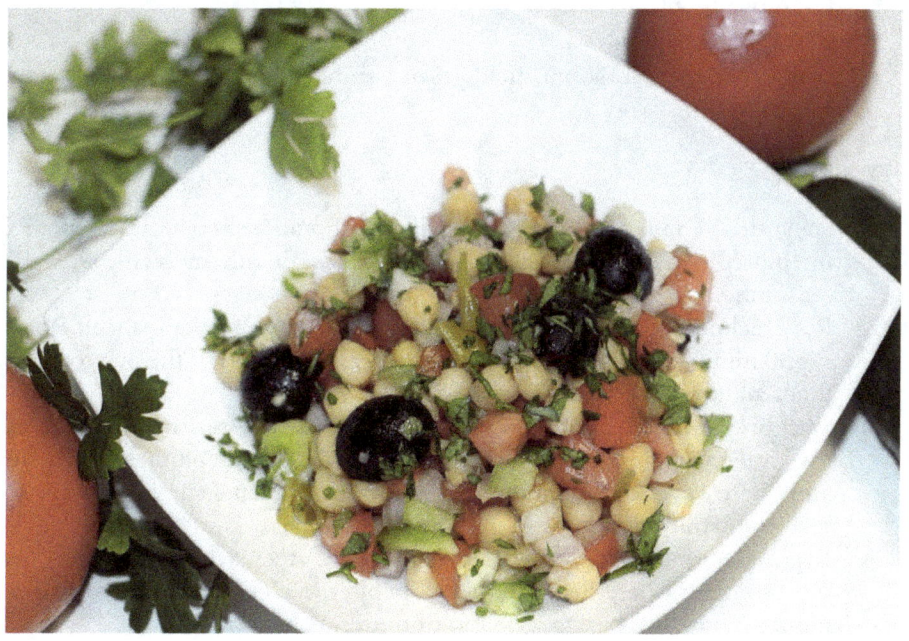

Ingredients

For the chickpeas

- Chickpeas (1 can, rinsed, drained, and skinned)
- Olive oil (1 tsp)
- Pinch of salt and pepper
- Dried basil (0.25 tsp)
- Garlic powder (0.25 tsp)

For the quinoa

- Quinoa (0.5 c.)
- Water (1 c.)

For the salad

- Bell pepper (1, color of choice, seeded, stemmed, and chopped to bite-sized bits)
- Cucumbers (2, peeled and chopped)
- Grape tomatoes (1 c., halved)
- Hummus (0.5 c.)
- Kalamata olives (0.5 c.)
- Lettuce (2 c. – can sub in field greens, spinach, kale, or any other leafy greens)

Instructions

1. Set your oven up to prepare for baking. It should be at 0400F. Then, mix the ingredients for the chickpeas together, coating them evenly with the seasoning.
2. Put chickpeas in single layer and put them onto the baking sheet. Roast for 30 minutes with an occasional mixing and rotation of the pan to allow them all to cook evenly. Allow them to cool.
3. Start preparing the quinoa and water in a microwave-safe bowl. Combine the water and quinoa and microwave, covered, for 4 minutes. Then stir and microwave for 2 minutes longer. Give it one final stir and leave it to rest in the microwave for another minute or two.
4. Begin assembling your salad. Begin with the greens at the bottom, then top with tomatoes, cucumbers, bell pepper, olives, chickpeas, and then quinoa. Finally, top with a dollop of hummus to serve

Vegan Mediterranean Pasta

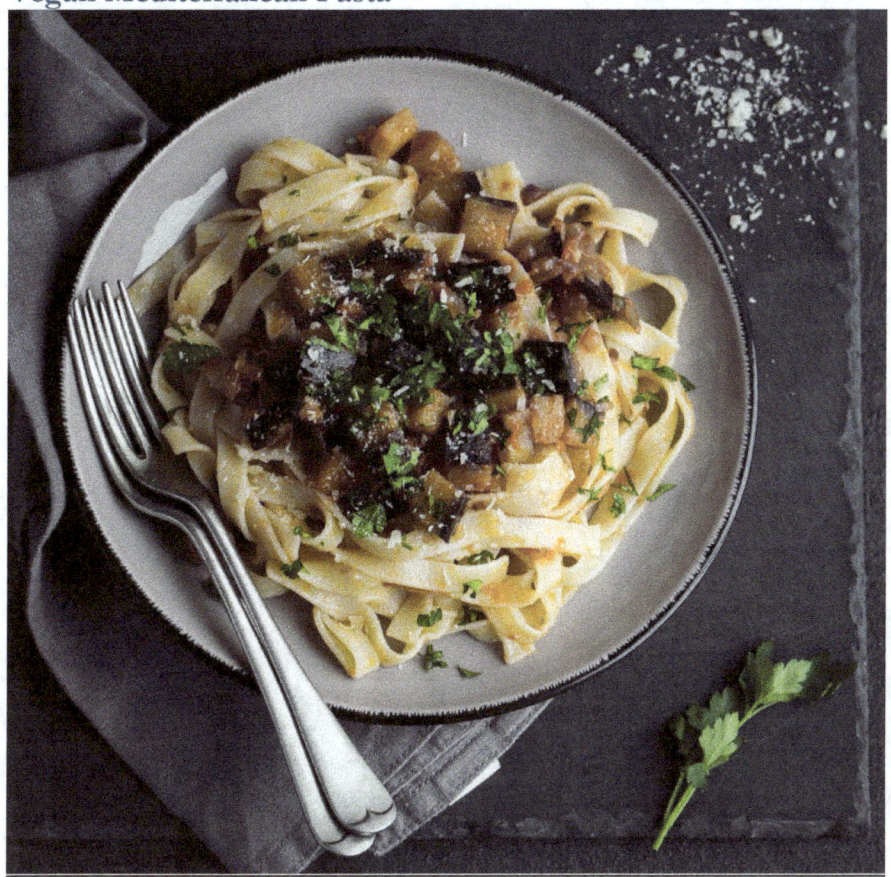

Ingredients

- Artichokes (0.5 c.)
- Basil leaves (0.25 c., torn)
- Garlic cloves (2-3 to taste, minced)
- Grape tomatoes (2 c., halved)
- Kalamata olives (10, pitted)
- Olive oil (1 Tbsp.)
- Pasta (8 oz.)
- Red pepper (0.25 tsp.)
- Salt and pepper to taste
- Spinach (4 c.)
- Tomato paste (4 Tbsp.)

- Vegetable broth (1 c.)

Instructions

1. Prepare your pasta based on the instructions provided. Keep 1 c. of the water for later use and then set the pasta aside.
2. While preparing your pasta, take the time to warm a large skillet with oil. Then, sauté your garlic and red pepper for 30 seconds or so. Combine in the tomato paste and cook for another minute. At that point, mix in your tomatoes, your seasoning, your artichokes and olives, and your broth. Let it cook until tomatoes start to break down.
3. Mix in the pasta to the tomato mixture. Let it cook another 2 minutes and add reserved pasta water if too dry.
4. Add in spinach and basil and cook until wilted.
5. Remove from heat and serve.

Vegetarian Zucchini Lasagna Rolls

Ingredients

- Basil (2 Tbsp., fresh)
- Egg (1, lightly beaten)
- Frozen spinach (10-ounce package, thawed and dried)
- Garlic (1 clove)
- Marinara sauce (0.75 c.)
- Olive oil (2 tsp)
- Parmesan cheese (3 Tbsp.)
- Pinch each of salt and pepper
- Ricotta (1.33 c.)
- Shredded mozzarella cheese (8 Tbsp.)
- Zucchini (2, trimmed)

Instructions

1. Prepare two baking sheets with cooking spray. Then set the oven to 425F.
2. Cut up your zucchini into strips lengthwise into 1/8 inch thick pieces. A mandolin will make this easier.
3. Prepare zucchini coated in oil with salt and pepper, then set up a flat layer across the bottom of the prepared pan.
4. Bake zucchini for 10 minutes until it begins to soften.
5. Mix together 2 Tbsp. mozzarella and 1 Tbsp. of parmesan. Then, in another bowl, combine egg, ricotta, spinach, garlic, and the remainder of the cheese. Toss in a pinch of salt and pepper and mix well.
6. Set up an 8-inch square casserole dish with 0.25 c. marinara spread across the bottom.
7. Take your zucchini that has been softened and begin to roll it. To do this, you will need to put 1 Tbsp. of ricotta mix at the bottom of your strip, then roll. Put the seam down in the marinara-covered bottom. Do this for all pieces of zucchini.
8. Cover the rolls with the remainder of your marinara sauce and top with the cheese mix.
9. Bake until bubbling, roughly 20 minutes. Rest for 5 minutes and top with basil.

Vegetarian Breakfast Sandwich

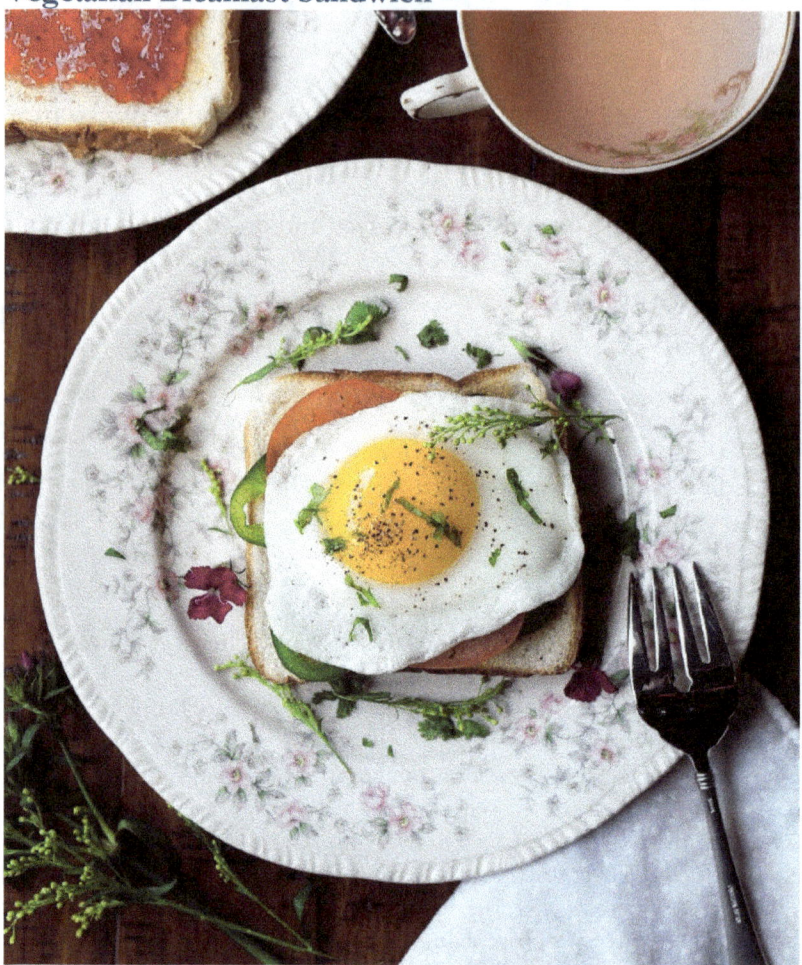

Ingredients

- Sandwich thins (2)
- Olive oil (2 Tbsp. + 1 tsp)
- Rosemary (1 Tbsp. fresh, or 0.5 tsp dried)
- Eggs (2)
- Spinach leaves (1 c.)
- Tomato (0.5, sliced thinly)
- Feta (2 Tbsp.)
- Pinch of salt and pepper

Instructions

1. Warm oven to 375F. Separate your sandwich thins and coat with olive oil. Bake for 5 minutes until beginning to crisp up.
2. Warm skillet with last tsp of olive oil. Break eggs into pan and cook until whites are set. Then, break the yolks and flip to finish cooking.
3. Put bottoms of the bread onto serving plates. Then, top with spinach, the tomato, one egg each, followed by the feta. Sprinkle with salt and pepper, then top with remaining bread.

Vegan Breakfast Toast

Ingredients

- Bread of choice (verify that it is vegan—2 slices)
- Spice blend of choice
- Arugula (handful)
- Tomato (1, cut into rounds)
- Chopped olives (1 Tbsp.)
- Cucumber (0.5, cut into rounds)
- Hummus (0.25 c.)

Instructions

1. Toast up your bread. Then spread the hummus across, season it, and top with all toppings split between the piece

Vegetarian Shakshouka

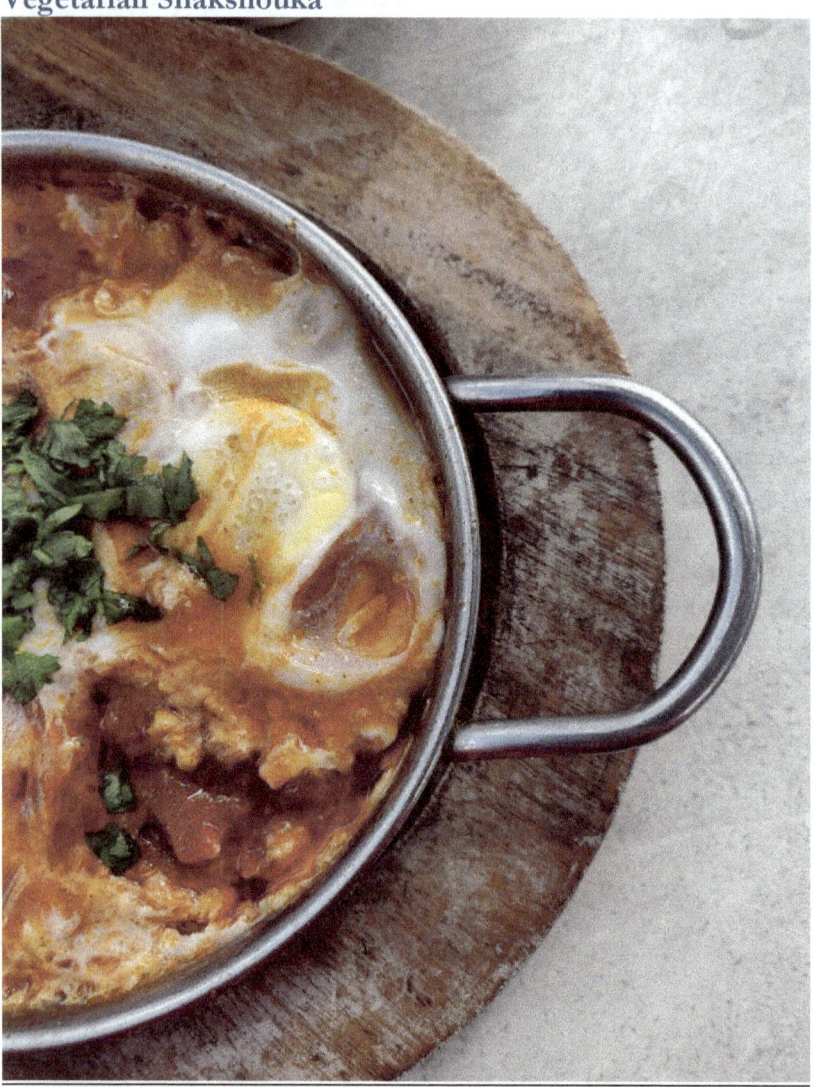

Ingredients

- Chopped parsley (1 Tbsp.)
- Diced Tomatoes (15 oz. can)
- Eggs (4)
- Garlic (2 cloves)
- Olive oil (2 Tbsp.)

- Onion (1—sliced)
- Red bell peppers (2, sliced thinly)
- Salt and pepper to taste
- Spicy harissa (1 tsp)
- Sugar (1 tsp)

Instructions

1. Warm oil in a cast iron pan. Sauté your peppers and onions until they have begun to soften, giving them a stir every now and then to prevent sticking. Add in the garlic for another minute.
2. Put in tomatoes, sugar, and harissa, leaving it to simmer for the next 7 minutes.
3. Season it to taste. Then, add in small indentations into the mixture in the pan, cracking an egg in each indentation that you make. Cover up the pot and allow it to cook until egg whites are done.

Cover with parsley and serve with bread.

www.ingramcontent.com/pod-product-compliance
Lightning Source LLC
LaVergne TN
LVHW020418070526
838199LV00055B/3660